THE SINETT SOLUTION

THE ULTIMATE BACKBRIDGE STRETCH BOOK

DR. TODD SINETT

Author of *Three Weeks to a Better Back*

EAST
END
PRESS

The BACKBRIDGE™ is a registered trademark of Dr. Todd Sinett.

THE ULTIMATE BACKBRIDGE STRETCH BOOK

Copyright © 2017 by Dr. Todd Sinett

Published by
EAST END PRESS
Bridgehampton, NY

ISBN: 978-0-9975304-1-4
Ebook ISBN: 978-0-9975304-2-1

FIRST EDITION

Book Design by Neuwirth & Associates
Cover Design by Dave Reidy

Manufactured in Canada

10 9 8 7 6 5 4 3 2 1

CONTENTS

Understanding Body Pain and the Growth of the Backbridge™

Dr. Todd Sinett's Story

In the early 1960s, my father, Dr. Sheldon Sinett, became a Chiropractor, not necessarily because of his deep desire to study the spine, but rather because a friend thought it was an up-and-coming profession. So my father graduated Chiropractic school even before there was a NY state license to practice and opened for business at my grandmother's house in Brooklyn, converting her front porch into an office. My grandmother would bake for the patients and my father would treat them, charging $10 for 3 treatments. My father would frequently tell me that when he started, no one knew what a Chiropractor was, and he attributed his success more my grandmother's baking skills than to his own chiropractic skills!

From his first office in my grandmother's house, my father learned a very important lesson, which he later taught to me: Always welcome a patient to your office like you would a guest to your living room. A photo of him with that quote is in my waiting room today.

My father quickly outgrew my grandmother's front porch and moved into a "real office" in Brooklyn. He would work from eight in the morning until eight at night, seeing tons of people. This went on for about 15 years until one day, he bent down to pick up a tennis ball and couldn't get back up. His back "went out", and after treating so many patients with severe pain, he found himself experiencing the same thing. He took a few days off from work to rest in bed, but the days turned into weeks, and the weeks turned into nine long months without any relief from his spasms and pain.

For those nine months, my father searched for answers to his own back problem. He never lost sight of how ironic it was that someone who made a living helping people with their back pain was suddenly completely debilitated from that same ailment. He went for endless treatments and consultations with every known profession, including his own, but nothing helped. A surgeon recommended exploratory surgery (never a good term), offering to open him up to see if they could find anything.

Hoping to find another option, he went to see a doctor in Detroit with the fortuitous name of Dr. George Goodheart. Dr. Goodheart asked one question that no one else had bothered to ask: *Why are you having the back spasms?* All the other doctors failed because they focused on treating the spasms rather than getting to the cause of the spasms. According to Dr. Goodheart, the answer, oddly enough, was that my father's diet, which consisted of sugar and caffeine, was upsetting his digestive system. Anything that can upset your digestive system, Dr Goodheart surmised, can then reflex and impact your muscular system, thus causing back spasms. My father's reaction to this was complete disbelief. But given the options to either change his diet or have exploratory surgery, he chose to change his diet. Dr. Goodheart treated him just a handful of times in conjunction with a complete change in his nutrition, and lo and behold,

my father was cured in just a few short weeks.

My father's life and my family's lives were changed forever. He dedicated his professional time to learning and expanding the teachings of Dr. Goodheart. Dr. Goodheart spoke of the "triad of health", or bringing one's body into balance on three different levels:

1. *structural, such as muscle and bones*
2. *diet and nutrition*
3. *emotions and stress*

Armed with this new knowledge and approach, my father became quite successful in treating thousands of patients, including many of the world's most famous people.

In 1995, I decided to join my father in practice after having my own pivotal experience. It was my sophomore year in college, and I was unsure of what to do with my life. We were on vacation in Aruba, and the local pediatrician had asked my father if he would examine a boy who was suffering from terrible, debilitating headaches. I went along with my father to the hospital and watched as he found that the boy's headaches were coming from an imbalance in his jaw and cranial bones. My father gave him one treatment, and the boy's headache went away. The next day, the boy's family came to the beach to bring my father money, which my father refused. The next day they came back with food–an offer that couldn't be turned away!

I knew from that day on that I would join my father and learn as much as I could to benefit as many people as possible. Everything that we did in our office, and that I continue to do, is to help people achieve the triad of health, or gain balance in their body, diet, and emotions. I had the great fortune to work with my dad for more than 15 years. We wrote a book together, *The Truth About Back Pain*, which was published in 2008 by Penguin after my father's death. The basic premise of the book is that we (as health professionals) are only looking at one-third of the causes of and treatments for back pain, and are essentially missing two-thirds of the information that we need to cure it. The role that diet and stress can play in back pain has been completely overlooked and ignored. The book went on to be printed in soft cover in a new edition that came out in 2014. Subsequently, I published a second book in 2015, *3 Weeks To A Better Back: Solutions for Healing the Structural, Nutritional, and Emotional Causes of Back Pain*, which investigates the principles more deeply and offers additional tools for self-help.

THE DEVELOPMENT OF THE BACKBRIDGE

Armed with my own inquisitive nature and a desire to cure the dominant physical causes that lead to back pain, I started to study the effects of how flexion, or too much forward hunch, and posture contributes. The benefits of extension therapy became quite intriguing to me, but it wasn't until I began working with a patient who happened to be an ESPN fitness model that I had my "aha" moment. She was the picture of health but was suffering terribly with neck and back pain. Her appearance and her symptoms just didn't match up. In taking her case history, she stated that she did thousands of sit-up and crunches on her fitness show. *Could these exercises be putting her body into too much forward hunch and be causing her pain?* I wondered. To test this theory I grabbed one of the big exercise balls we had in our therapy room and had her lay on her back to stretch over it. To her surprise and mine, after stretching over the ball for a few minutes she felt significantly better. I then took the ball and went to show my father what I had discovered. He proceeded to lie over the ball—only to fall off of it!

Off to the drawing board I went. I wanted to design a product that was more stable and put extension into one's spine in a gradual and safe manner. After years of tinkering, I finally perfected it and created a product called the Backbridge. With its different levels, the Backbridge allows anyone to use it comfortably by progressively undoing all of the forward hunch that our body gets throughout the day.

The amazing thing about my discovery was that I realized that athletes and super fit people were not the only ones suffering from back pain caused by too much flexion. The average person, and even the out-of-shape ones, were as well. While the athlete may have developed their imbalance from exercise that puts too much flexion into the body, the average person was developing theirs from excessive amounts of sitting or too much forward pull from weight gain, etc. The commonality across all ages and all demographics was too much forward hunch, or flexion, creating core imbalance which resulted in back pain.

By creating my Backbridge, I was able to help hundreds, if not thousands of my patients, who continued to be astounded by the results. Patients started getting the Backbridges for their family members and friends, and it wasn't long before I was shipping them to movie sets and musicians were taking them on tour. I like to think of the Backbridge as the Invisalign® for the spine. The Backbridge is also a great support for your desk chair or car seat.

The Ultimate Backbridge Stretch Book

After creating the Backbridge, I continually experimented on how else it could be of help. I first started doing back stretches with the Backbridge, but then I gave it to fitness trainers, yoga instructors, fellow chiropractors and physical therapists, and the possibilities expanded exponentially from there. The result is *The Ultimate Backbridge Stretch Book*. By utilizing the Backbridge, you are able to combine health and fitness and fix your posture, train your core and dramatically improve your flexibility. This book is designed to give you several stretching options:

- ▶ A full-body stretch routine, which is a great daily practice that can be done in just 15 minutes, allowing you to make it part of your everyday life.

- ▶ A focused back stretch plan, intended to counteract the effects of flexion in our day and is great for anyone suffering from back pain of any kind.

- ▶ Targeting your tight spots, which allows you to identify your area of tightness and flip to stretches that will loosen that specific area.

- ▶ Tandem or partner stretching to increase the intensity of a stretch while maintaining proper form.

- ▶ Balance and proprioception exercises to help you stabilize your body and avoid injury.

- ▶ Backbridge Yoga, which takes traditional yoga poses and adds the Backbridge, giving you greater range of motion and allowing you to modify and grow in your yoga practice.

We'll learn about each muscle group as we go and how the Backbridge can enhance the stretches you can do for every part of your body.

RECLAIM YOUR FLEXIBILITY WITH THE BACKBRIDGE

Aging, exercise, and the daily stressors and baggage of life affect our body in many ways, most of which manifest in soreness, tightness or other feelings of pain. Even activities that don't seem harmful, like sitting, can put stress on our bodies and allow them to become stiff. There have even been studies that have called sitting "the new smoking." While we may not be able to control the amount of hours that we have to sit (because of our jobs and lives), this book can help you counteract a lot of the harmful effects caused by sitting and other daily activities. Stretching is a gentle exercise that should be done daily to help you loosen up stiff and tender muscles, relieve discomfort, and regain the flexibility you had as a child. It can even lengthen your life.

Why is it important to reclaim your flexibility? Our flexibility affects our ability to bend and move and impacts our overall vitality. In order to be truly healthy and fit, you need to have a balance of three fitness factors: 1) endurance, 2) strength, and 3) flexibility. As a doctor, I have seen way too many patients and athletes who have more than adequate strength and aerobic function, but who are severely lacking flexibility.

The Benefits of Improved Flexibility

1. Better posture

Having great flexibility means you'll also be able to stand up straighter, walk farther, and do more things with less pain. As we age, our joints and muscles stiffen, making it more difficult to perform various tasks, such as bending over, walking up steps and even sitting.

2. Improved coordination prevents injury

Improved flexibility allows us to have better balance and coordination. Better balance and coordination means fewer falls.

3. Improved Blood Circulation

Blood is pumped back to your heart through your veins by the squeezing and relaxing of skeletal muscles. Stretching helps relax your muscles, allowing circulation to improve. This has obvious benefits such as increased oxygen delivery, reduction in cramping, and an increased capacity for performance. In other words, better flexibility leads to better endurance and better recovery.

The Backbridge for Improved Flexibility

In 2008 I created the Backbridge to help people correct core imbalance and back pain. The vast majority of us are suffering from core imbalance caused by too much forward hunch. This flexion is brought on by our aging process, improper exercise practices, as well as being slumped forward all day in front of computers, while commuting, texting on mobile devices, or anything else we may do while we are sitting with poor posture. As I continued to help people with their back pain, core imbalance, and spinal flexibility, I realized the Backbridge doesn't just return flexibility to your spine, it returns flexibility to your entire body.

The Backbridge is the perfect tool to help you achieve improved flexibility for two main reasons:

1. Its arched, contoured design maximizes a muscle's isolation, resulting in a deeper, better stretch.

2. Its interlocking, stackable levels allow you to alter the intensity of any stretch.
When you stretch at your own level of flexibility, you prevent injuries and discomfort from over-stretching. In some stretches, the highest level of the Backbridge (level 5) will allow for the

easiest stretch by limiting the amount of stretch and/or range of motion, while using level 5 in other stretches will create the maximum amount of stretch. (This will be noted throughout the book so you can determine how to increase or decrease the stretch.) As you improve your flexibility, you will be able to increase the stretch factor just by adding or removing levels. Without the Backbridge, stretches are static and essentially always the same. You wouldn't want to continually lift the same amount of weight or always do the same amount of aerobic exercise because your strength and endurance will plateau. So why would you always want to stretch the same? Being able to deepen your stretches allows your body to become stronger and more flexible, and the Backbridge allows you to progress gradually and safely.

Stretching Tips

As we move through this book, here are tips to remember to help you maximize the benefits of stretching:

1. **The golden rule: Do not bounce while stretching.** Find a comfortable position and remain static in your stretch.

2. **Move slowly.** It's not a race, so ease into each stretch to reduce the risk of over-stretching and subsequent injury.

3. **Stretch often.** Stretching increases the elasticity of your muscles, but you can't do it all in one 15 minute stretching workout. Stretching should be done frequently. Remember, one stretch won't make you flexible, just like going on one run won't make you aerobically fit. Make stretching a consistent part of your fitness routine.

4. **Breathe.** The key is to relax so you can achieve a better stretch. Remembering to breathe allows you to let go of the stress.

5. **It shouldn't be painful.** You shouldn't be grimacing in pain while stretching. Make sure to listen to your body and stay within your limits. While you should approach your boundaries, only do what you're actually capable of doing. Remember, if it hurts, don't do it. This is your body telling you to stop. A stretch should be enjoyable!

DO NOT START NEW EXERCISE/STRETCH ROUTINE WITHOUT CONSULTING A PHYSICIAN.

THE ULTIMATE BACKBRIDGE STRETCH BOOK

1

Full Body Stretch Routine with the Backbridge

This stretch routine is something I do just about every day. It helps me start my day loose, limber and energized. Ideally, this whole routine can be done in about 15-20 minutes, which makes it easy to fit into your daily life.

Make sure to do each stretch on both sides of your body when it applies, holding each stretch for about 20 seconds unless otherwise noted. If you have more time, feel free to do each stretch longer or add stretches to the routine. If you are pressed for time, you can also alternate stretch days of upper and lower extremity; however, I recommend to always include the six stretches in Group 1 (the full body warm-up stretches) in any routine. How much time you allocate to stretching is completely up to you, but consistency is key. Pick a routine that works for you so that you can continue stretching with your Backbridge for the rest of your life. Remember, maintaining good flexibility is vital to one's health!

GROUP 1

FULL BODY WARM-UP

Backbridge Extension

This stretch is why I created the Backbridge. It puts much needed extension into one's spine while counteracting all of the forward hunch that we do all day. It extends the spine, opens up the chest and shoulders, and realigns your posture. It is proven to rid your body of back pain caused by postural imbalances.

To do the stretch, sit at the base of the Backbridge. Lie back so that the highest point of the Backbridge is between your shoulder blades and your head is touching the floor. Rest your arms on the ground behind your head and hold this stretch for 2 minutes. You can do this stretch with your legs extended or your knees bent. Level 1 is the easiest and 5 is the hardest. Pick a level that is most comfortable for you. It should feel like a good stretch. After a few weeks, slowly progress to the next level.

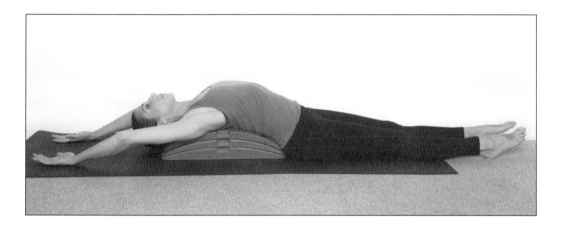

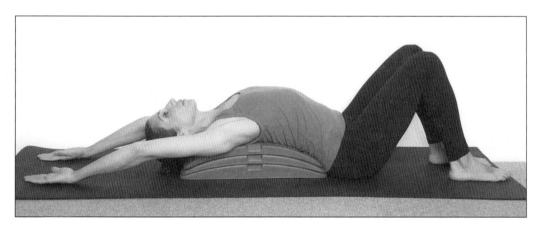

Spinal Stretch

Lie on your back, placing the Backbridge under your knees. The level doesn't affect the stretch here, so choose which feels most comfortable. Reach your arms behind you (over your head along the ground) to lengthen the spine.

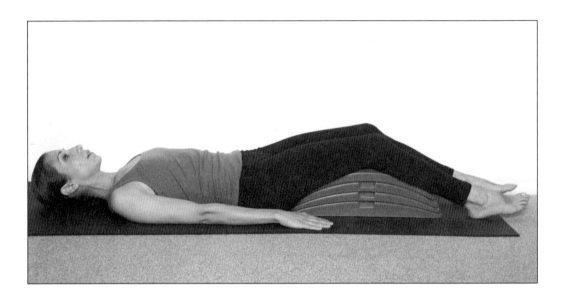

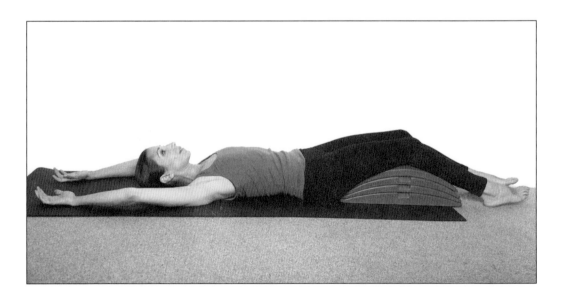

Side Lying Stretch

Lie on your side and stretch over the Backbridge so that the highest point of the Backbridge is at your rib cage. With your bottom hand, grab the wrist of your top hand and extend your arms overhead along the ground. As you progress, add more levels of the Backbridge to increase the stretch and loosen up your side muscles (*latissimus dorsi*). Switch sides and repeat.

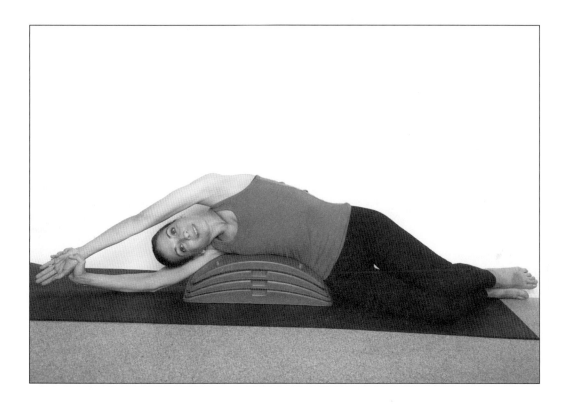

Side Lying Chest Stretch

While side lying on the Backbridge, extend your upper arm and then reach back so that your chest opens to the ceiling. Angle this arm in slightly different directions to stretch different fibers of your pectoral (chest) muscles. Switch sides and repeat.

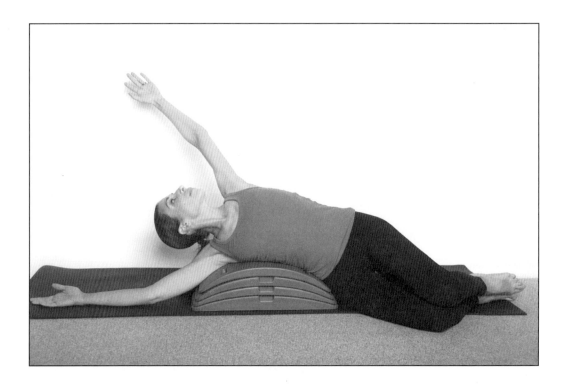

Abdominal Stretch (Cobra)

Lie face down over the Backbridge and place your hands in front of you. Do half a push up so that your upper torso is elevated, but your pelvis still has contact with the Backbridge. Focus straight ahead of you to maintain length in your neck (avoid crunching in the back of the neck). Hold for a count of five, then slowly lower yourself down and repeat. This stretch really works your lumbar extenders and lower back while stretching and lengthening the core (abdominals). The higher the level of the Backbridge you use, the easier the stretch will be.

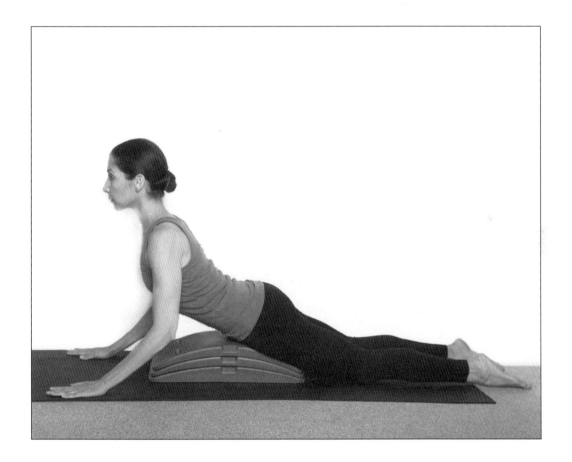

Reclining Twist

Place the Backbridge about 12 inches to the side of your hips. Extend your arms to the side in a "T," keeping your shoulders flat on the mat, and bring one knee towards your chest. With your other leg flat on the mat, pull your bent knee across your torso, placing it on the Backbridge. Hold the stretch and repeat on the opposite side. Try different levels of the Backbridge to find which is most comfortable for you (level 1 is the hardest.) If you can comfortably rest on level 1, try bringing your knee to the ground. The key to this stretch is keeping both of your shoulders on the mat.

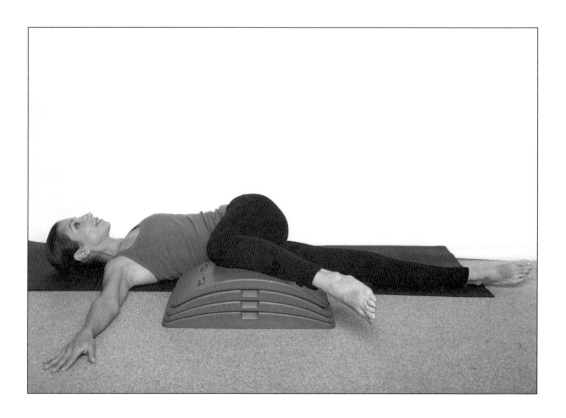

GROUP 2

LOWER EXTREMITY

Knees To Chest Stretch

For a low back stretch, place your buttocks on the highest point of the Backbridge and lay back on the mat. Wrap your hands behind your knees and gently pull your knees to your chest while reaching and lengthening your tailbone down towards the Backbridge. Hold for a few seconds. If you have trouble wrapping your hands around your knees, you can place them behind your legs on the backs of your thighs. The higher level of the Backbridge you use in this posture, the more intense the stretch.

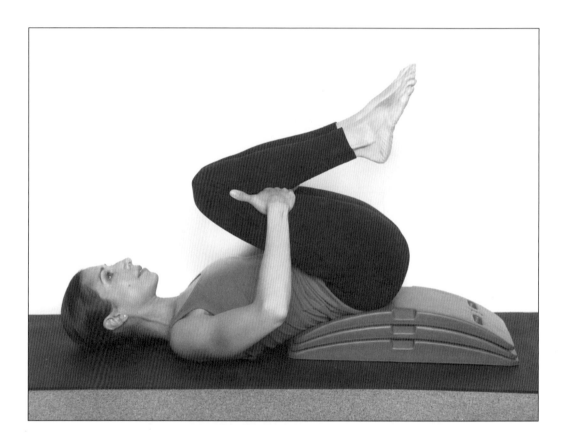

Single Knee To Chest Stretch

Set up like the Knee to Chest Stretch, but pull one leg toward your chest and extend the opposite leg over the Backbridge and along the mat. (For a less intense stretch, you may also keep this leg bent if it is more comfortable on your low back or hip flexor.) By gently angling the knee inward or outward, you will stretch different parts of your hip flexors. Switch legs and repeat.

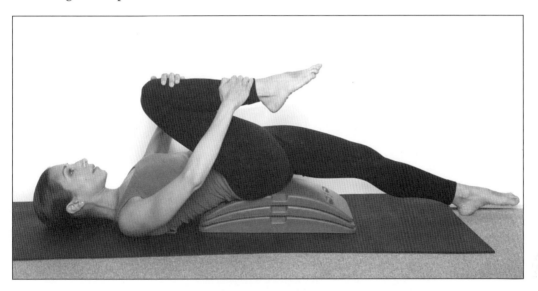

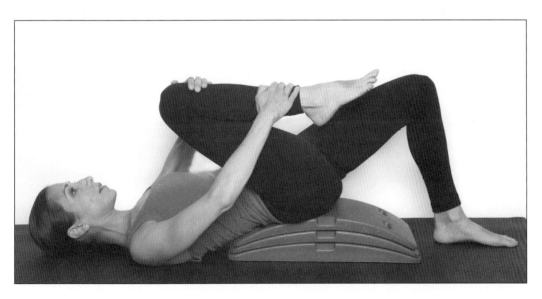

Piriformis and Outer Hip Stretch (Figure 4)

Place your buttocks on the highest point of the Backbridge and lie back on the mat. With both knees bent, cross one leg over the other. Wrap your hands behind your uncrossed leg (or bottom knee) and gently pull towards you. Keep the foot of your crossed leg flexed to protect the knee. Switch legs and repeat.

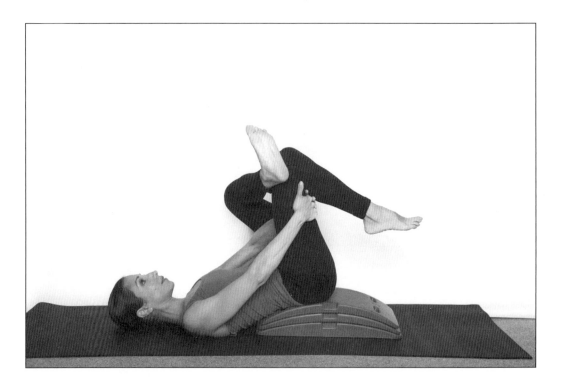

Hamstring Stretch (With Strap)

Sit on the highest point of the Backbridge and lie back on the mat. Bring one leg toward your chest and place the stretch strap around your foot just below the ball of your big toe, making sure the strap is flat. Extend your leg straight up above your hip, keeping your other leg extended over the Backbridge and down along the mat. If this is uncomfortable, it is okay to keep your bottom leg bent as pictured below. Gently pull the strap down and back towards your head to increase the stretch in your hamstring. Make sure to keep your leg and knee as straight as possible without locking, or hyperextending, your knee while doing this stretch. The higher the level of the Backbridge you use, the greater the stretch will be. Switch legs and repeat.

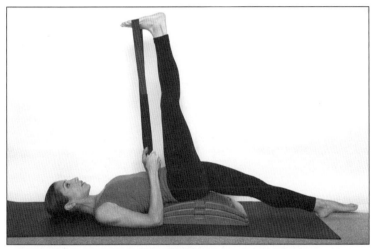

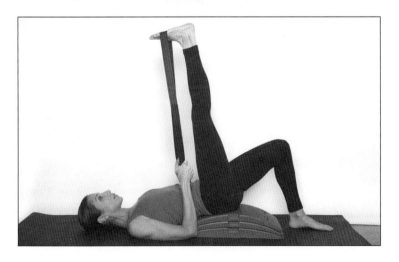

IT Band (iliotibial band) Stretch (With Strap)

Set up like the previous hamstring stretch and pull the stretch strap across your body. You should feel this stretch through your hip and along the outside of your thigh. Switch legs and repeat.

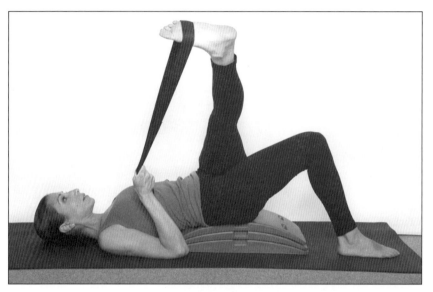

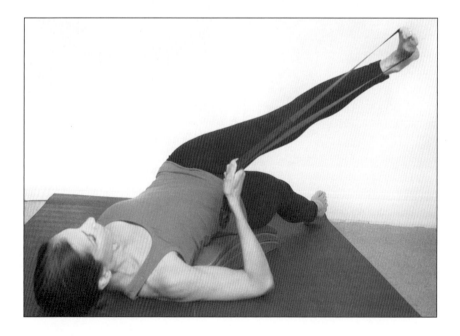

Hip Adductors (Inner Thigh) Stretch (With Strap)

Using the same setup as the previous stretches, pull your leg away from your body while maintaining contact on the Backbridge. You may want to bend the opposite leg, placing your foot on the mat for leverage. You will feel this stretch through the inner part of your thigh and groin. Switch legs and repeat.

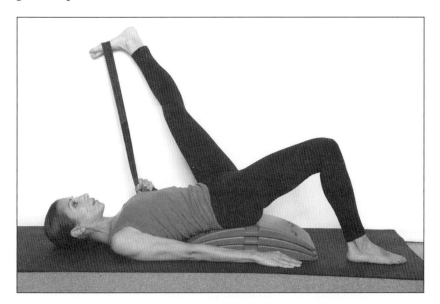

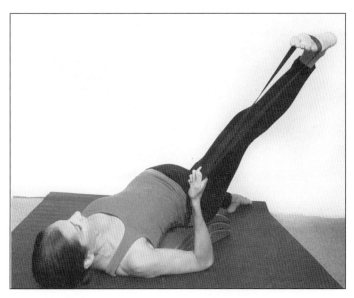

Inner Thigh and Groin Stretch

Sit in a cross-legged position on the Backbridge, placing your ankles in front of one another with the tops of your feet on the mat and your hands on your knees. Feel a gentle opening in your thighs, hips, and groin. Hold for a count of five, then switch the cross of the ankles.

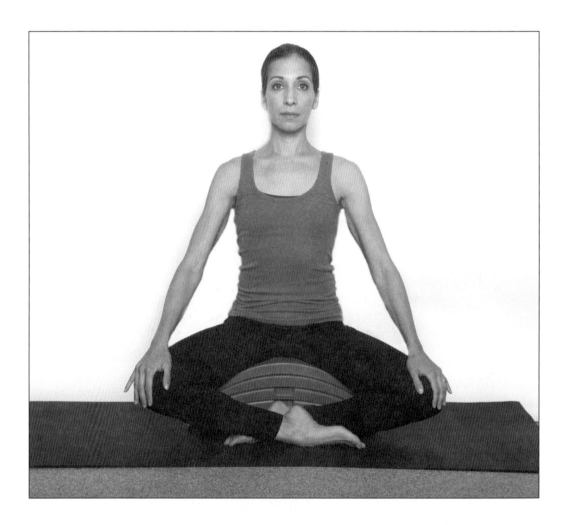

Inner Thigh and Groin Stretch (Butterfly)

Sit on the Backbridge and pull your feet in as close as possible. Place the soles of the feet together, letting the knees slowly drop open towards the mat. You can gently push down on your thighs with your elbows or on your lower legs with your forearms to increase the stretch. Using higher levels of the Backbridge will help people with tight hips by allowing your knees to drop open, similar to sitting on a block or blanket in yoga. As always, listen to your body and find the level that is best for you.

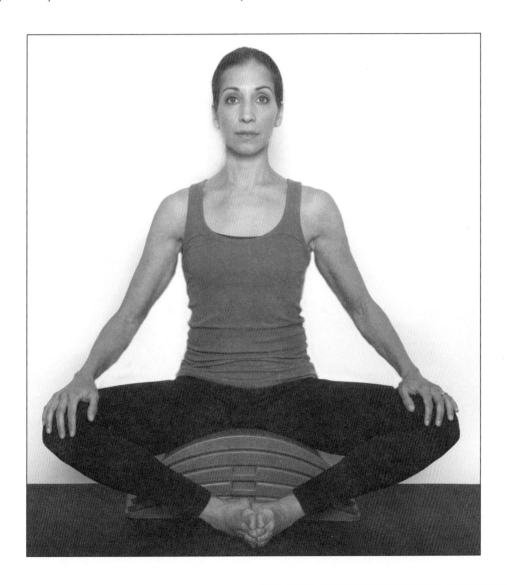

Lower Latissmus and Lumbar Rotator (Low back) Stretches

Sit on the Backbridge and spread your legs in a "V" position. Facing forward, bend your torso over to the right, sliding your right arm down your right leg. Raise your left arm over your head, so that your upper arm is next to your ear. Keep your palm open and facing the floor. Rotate your torso and head slowly towards the ceiling to open the chest, feeling the stretch in your lower back.

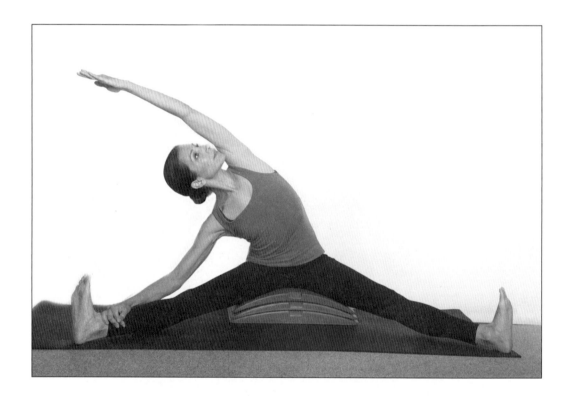

From the last stretch, bend your right arm and place your right hand on your right hip. Rotate your torso and head to face down, so that you are looking at your right knee. Your left arm should remain straight with palm down, parallel to floor.

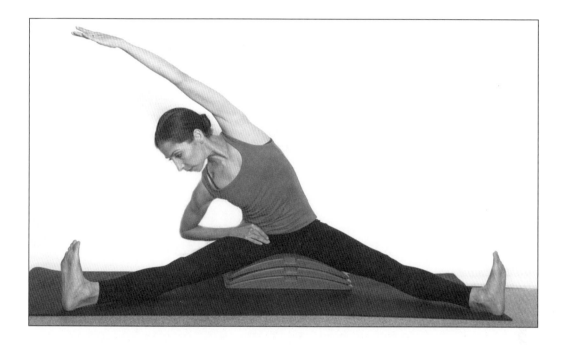

Still sitting in a split position, keep your torso rotated down and with both hands, reach for your right foot. Repeat all three of these stretches on left side.

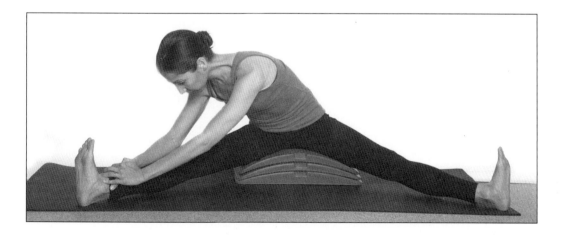

Lower Back and Groin Stretch

Sit on the Backbridge with legs spread in a "V." Keep your back as straight as possible and hinge at hips, bringing your forearms towards the mat.

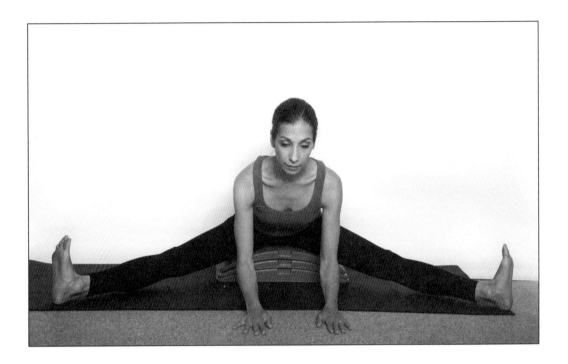

Quadriceps Stretch

Place the front of your right thigh just above the knee on the Backbridge and bring your left leg forward in a lunge position (keeping the knee bent at a 90 degree angle), bending your right knee to bring your foot closer to your buttocks, reach back with your right hand and hold your ankle or the top of your foot, slowly leaning forward. Repeat on left side. The higher the level of the Backbridge you use, the greater the stretch you will feel.

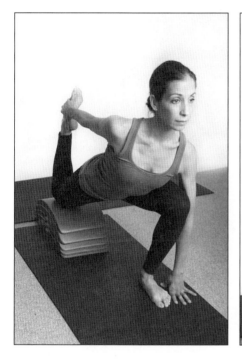 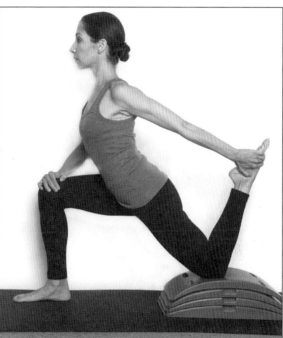

Hip Flexor Stretch

Start in the same position as the Quadriceps Stretch and then lower your front leg to the floor so that your shin and the top of your foot are resting on the mat. Lean forward and rest on your forearm. Flex or point your toe to alter the stretch. Repeat with opposite leg.

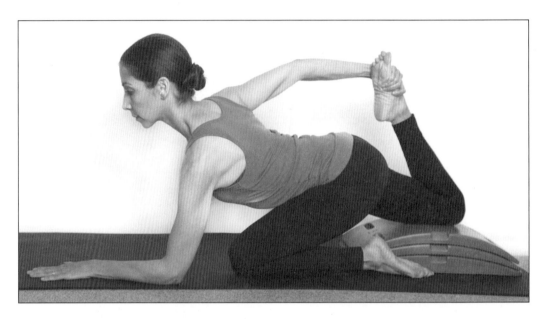

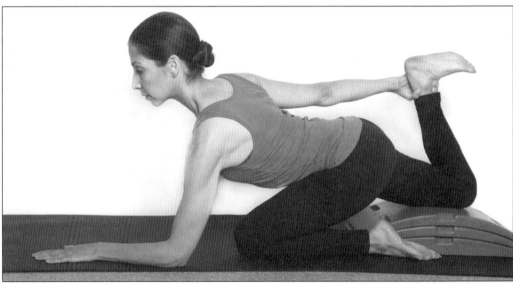

Calf Stretches

Using level 1 or 2 of the Backbridge (optimal height to engage the calf muscles), place your heels on the mat and your toes on the end of the Backbridge. Then stand on the side of the Backbridge and lower down one heel toward the mat, stretching that calf while your other foot remains flat. Repeat with both legs.

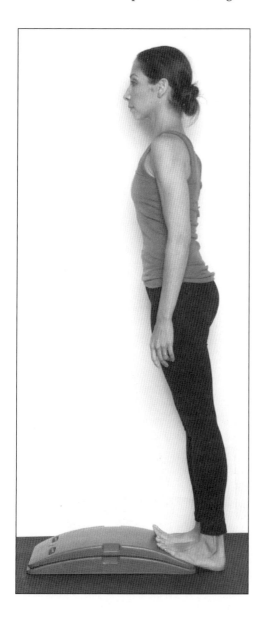
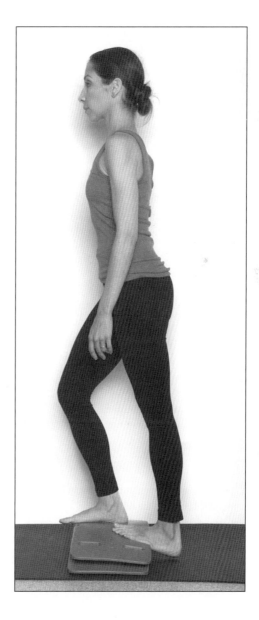

Ankle Stretches

Using levels 1 or 2 of the Backbridge, stretch out your ankle in all directions by turning your foot in and out and placing the top of your foot on the Backbridge. You can think about rotating your ankle around the face of a clock, pausing "on the hour." Reverse direction. Repeat on other ankle.

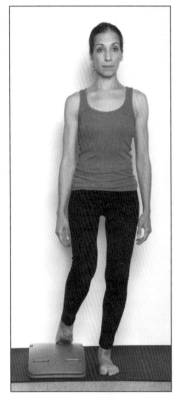
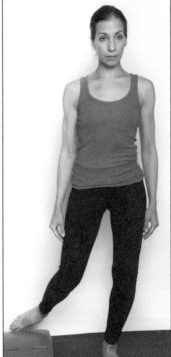
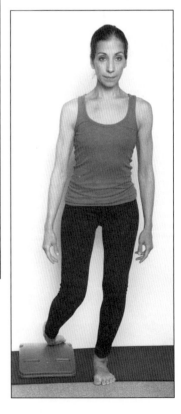

GROUP 3

UPPER EXTREMITY

Shoulder and Torso Stretch

Sitting on your knees, place your forearms on the Backbridge, interlock your fingers and lie forward as much as possible with your head between your upper arms. Leaning back, try to bring your buttocks to your heels. This will open up your shoulders and chest.

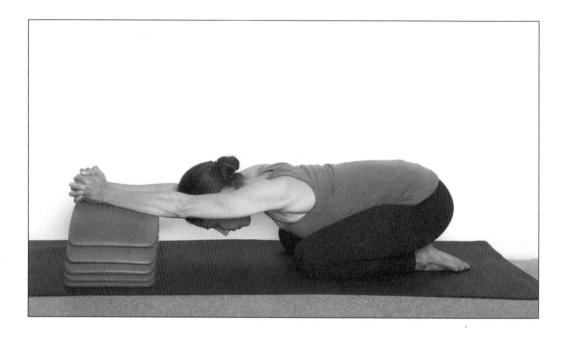

Shoulder and Torso Stretch with Twist

Sitting back on your knees, interlock your hands and lie forward so that your fists rest on the Backbridge. Twist your arms so that one hand rolls on top of other. Hold and then repeat on other side, switching your hands and twisting in the opposite direction.

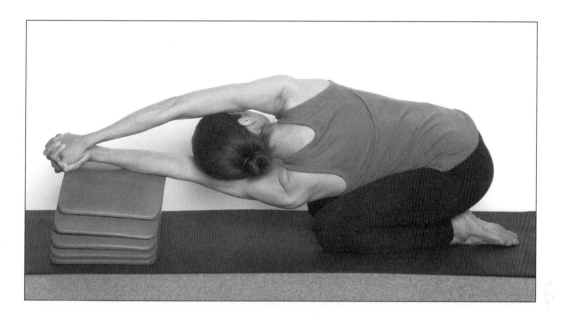

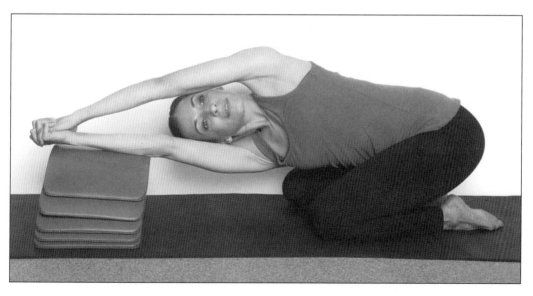

Shoulder Stretch with Intercrossed Arms

Sit back on your knees, straighten your arms, turn palms face up, and cross arms at the elbows. Lean forward so that your arms rest on the Backbridge and your head rests on your upper arms. Hold and then repeat, re-crossing arms with your opposite arm on top. You can try this same stretch with palms facing down for a slightly different sensation.

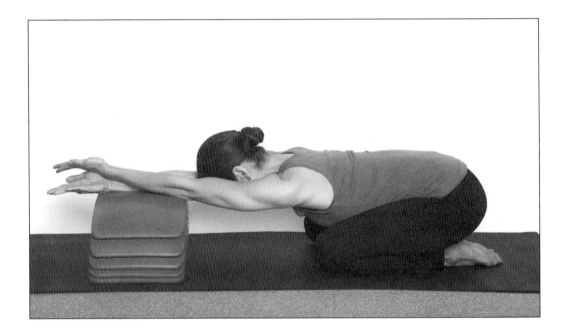

Post Deltoid Stretch (Thread The Needle)

While kneeling, place one arm face down on the Backbridge. Bring your other arm under and across your body, laying it on the mat, palm up. Try to keep your hips directly above your knees. Switch sides and repeat.

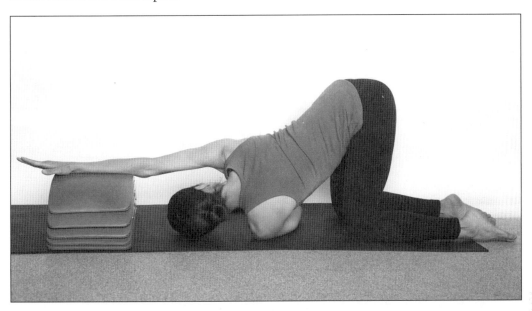

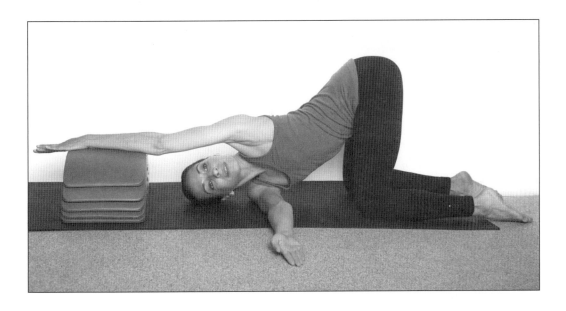

Shoulder and Triceps Stretch

While in the kneeling position, place your elbows on the Backbridge with arms bent at 90 degrees and palms together over your head.

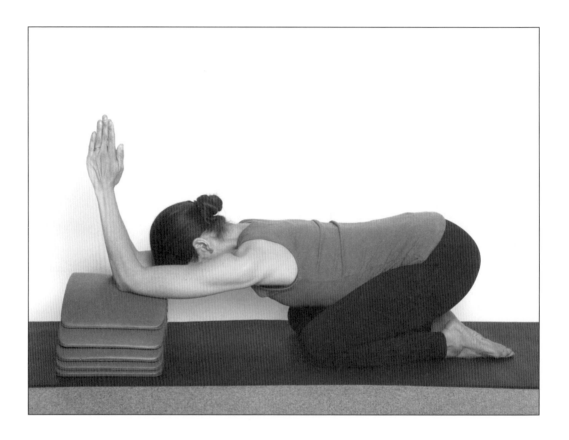

Pectoralis and Latissimus Dorsi (Lats) Stretches

In a kneeling position, extend one arm and shoulder face up on the Backbridge while your opposite arm reaches up to the ceiling. Hold and then switch arms.

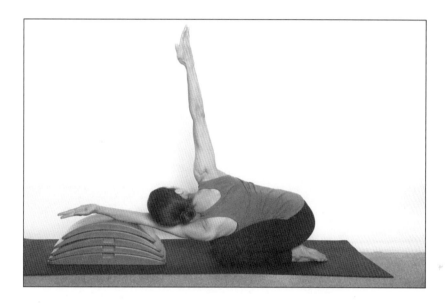

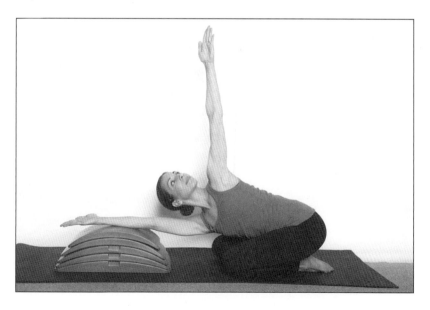

Posterior Deltoids, Lats and Serratus (Shoulder) Stretches

Lying face down on the mat, place one arm and shoulder on the Backbridge and your other arm in front of you, flat on the floor next to it. Rotate your palm down and hold. Rotate your thumb up and hold. Rotate your palm up and hold. Rotating the placement of your hand on the Backbridge will alter the stretch, so you will feel the pull on the sides and backs of your shoulder. Switch arms and repeat.

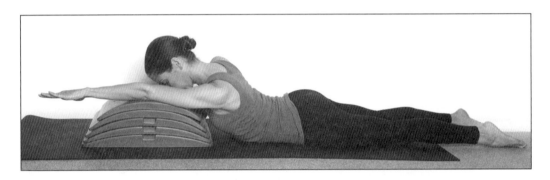

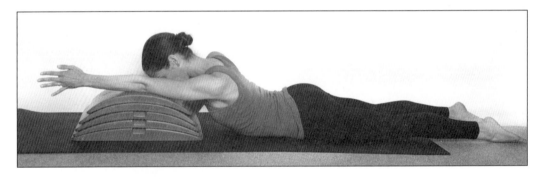

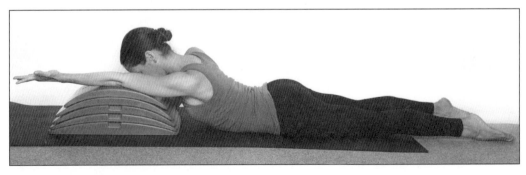

Wrist and Forearm Stretches

Make two fists and lay the backside of your hands flat on the Backbridge, fists touching.

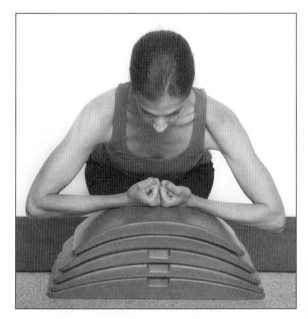

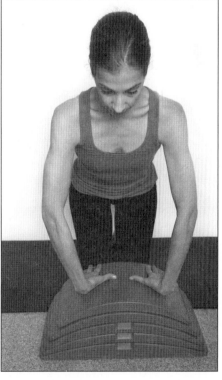

Lie both wrists on the Backbridge, palms up with your fingers facing towards you.

Place the back side of both wrists on the Backbridge with your thumbs turned out.

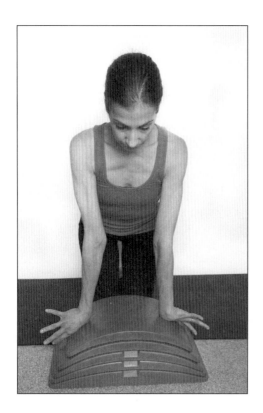
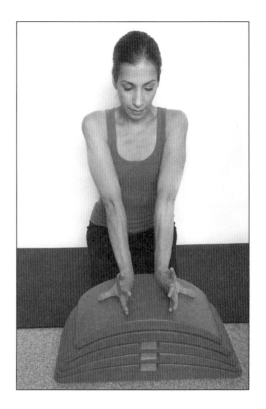

Place your wrists on the Backbridge, with your fingers pointing towards each other and your palms facing up. Lean into the stretch.

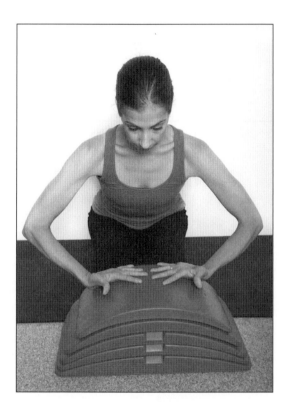
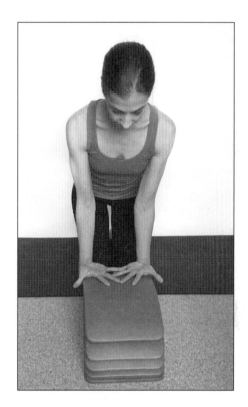

Thumb Stretches

Place your thumbs on the edge of the Backbridge and gently push down.

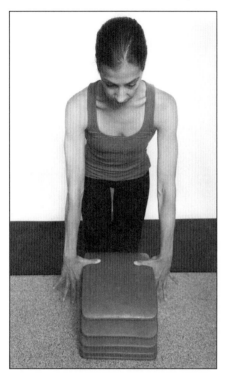

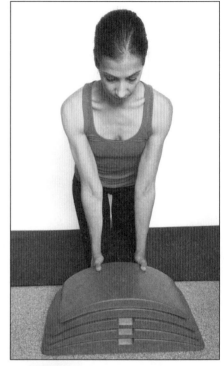

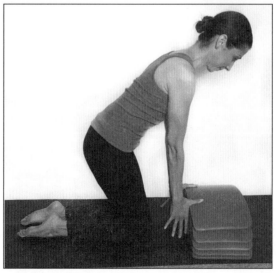

The Top 10 Stretches For a Better Back

As a chiropractor and the author of *3 Weeks to a Better Back*, I know people are always complaining about back pain and looking for good back stretches. These ten back stretches will realign your spine and help correct postural imbalances that can be the underlying source of common back pain. While most of them are included in the full body stretch routine, it is important to note which stretches specifically improve back flexibility. The better your spinal alignment, the better your posture and flexibility, and the better your back will be—not to mention your overall quality of life! Remember, these stretches are not only intended to help you recover from back pain, but to prevent it as well.

BACK STRETCH PROTOCOL

1. Backbridge Extension

Sit at the base of the Backbridge. Lie back so that the highest point of the Backbridge is between your shoulder blades and your head is touching the floor. Rest your arms on the ground behind your head and hold this stretch for 2 minutes. You can do this stretch with your legs extended or your knees bent. Level 1 is the easiest and 5 is the hardest. Pick a level that is most comfortable for you. It should feel like a good stretch. After a few weeks, slowly progress to the next level.

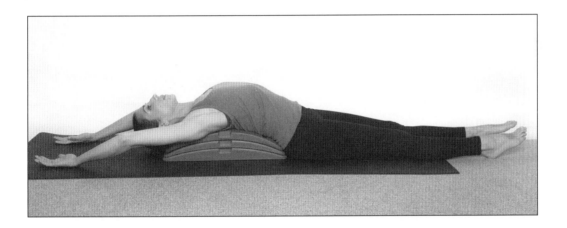

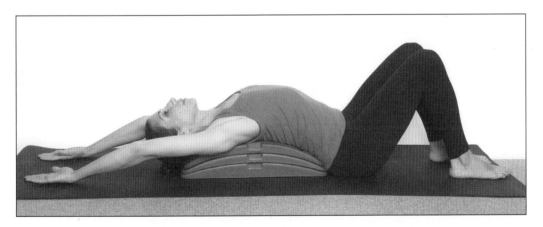

2. Spinal Stretch

Lie on your back, placing the Backbridge under your knees. The level doesn't affect the stretch here, so choose which feels most comfortable. Reach your arms over head to lengthen the spine.

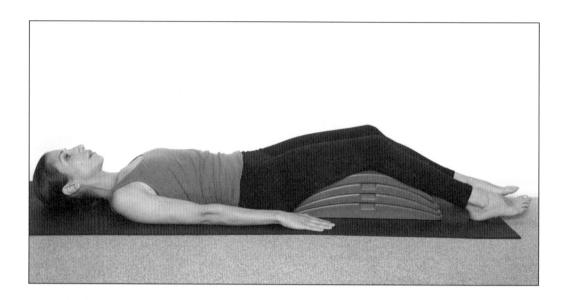

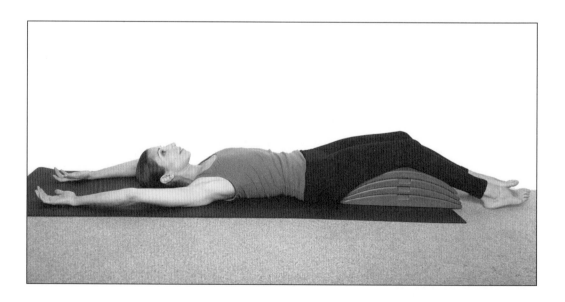

3. Side Lying Stretch

Lie on your side and stretch over the Backbridge so that the highest point of the Backbridge is at your rib cage. With your bottom hand, grab the wrist of your top hand and extend your arms overhead along the ground. As you progress, add more levels of the Backbridge to increase the stretch and loosen up your side muscles (*latissimus dorsi*). Switch sides and repeat.

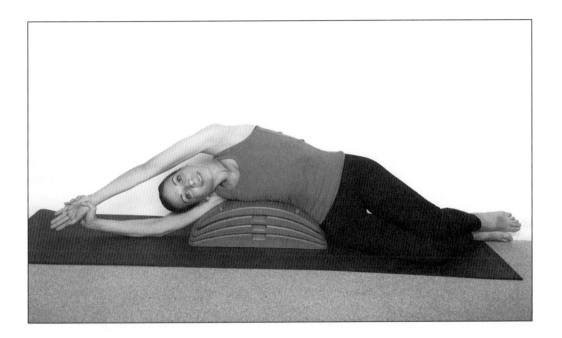

4. Abdominal Stretch (Cobra)

Lie face down over the Backbridge and place your hands in front of you. Do half a push up so that your upper torso is elevated, but your pelvis still has contact with the Backbridge. Focus straight ahead of you to maintain length in your neck (avoid crunching the back of the neck). Hold for a count of five, then slowly lower yourself down and repeat. This stretch really works your lumbar extenders and lower back while stretching and lengthening the core (abdominals). The higher the level of the Backbridge you use, the easier the stretch will be.

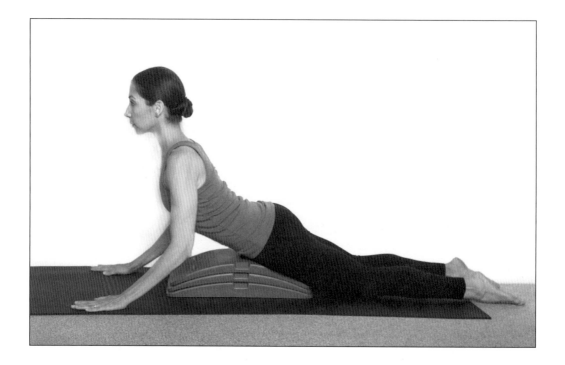

5. Reclining Twist

Place the Backbridge about 12 inches to the side of your hips. Extend your arms in a "T", keeping your shoulders flat on the mat, and bring one knee towards your chest. With your other leg flat on the mat, pull your bent knee over your torso, placing it on the Backbridge. Hold the stretch and repeat on the opposite side. Try different levels of the Backbridge to find which is most comfortable for you (level 1 is the hardest.) If you can comfortably rest on level 1, try bringing your knee to the ground. The key to this stretch is keeping both of your shoulders on the mat. Repeat on the opposite side.

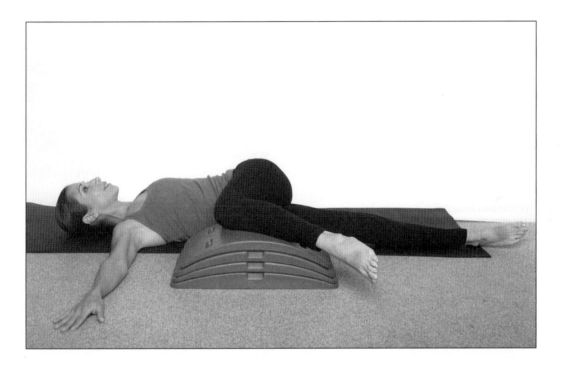

6. Knees To Chest Stretch

For a low back stretch, place your buttocks on the highest point of the Backbridge and lay back on the mat. Wrap your hands behind your knees and gently pull your knees to your chest while reaching and lengthening your tailbone down towards the Backbridge. Hold for a few seconds. If you have trouble wrapping your hands around your knees, you can place them behind your legs on the back of your thighs. The higher level of the Backbridge you use in this posture, the more intense the stretch.

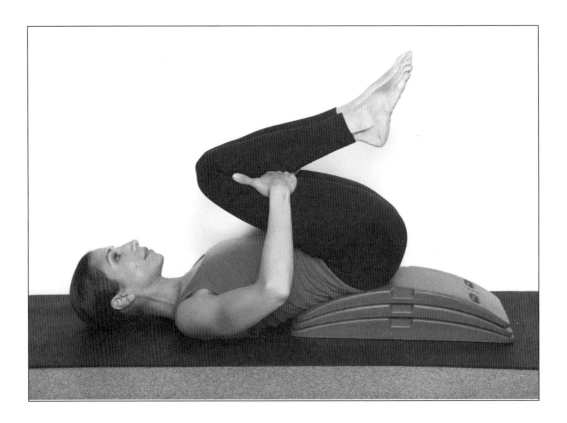

7. Single Knee to Chest Stretch

Set up like the Knee to Chest stretch, but pull one leg toward your chest and extend the opposite leg over the Backbridge and along the mat. By gently angling the knee inward or outward, you will stretch different parts of your hip flexors. Switch legs and repeat.

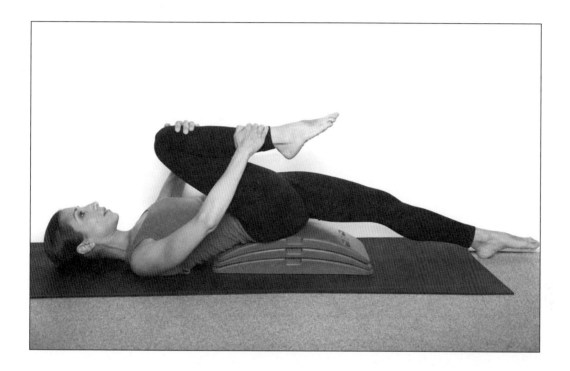

8. Piriformis and Outer Hip Stretch (Figure 4)

Place your buttocks on the highest point of the Backbridge and lie back on the mat. With both knees bent, cross one leg over the other. Wrap your hands behind your uncrossed leg (or bottom knee) and gently pull towards you. Keep the foot of the crossed leg flexed to protect your knee. Switch legs and repeat.

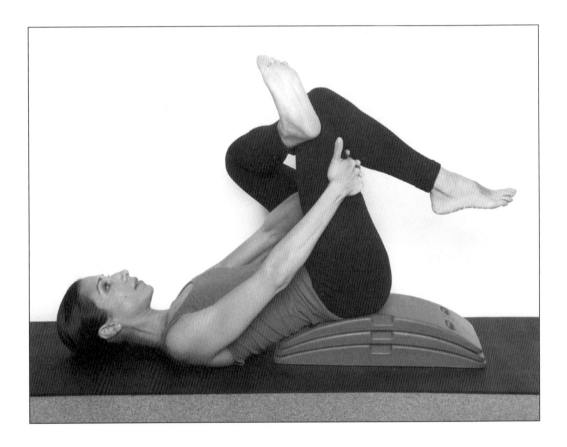

9. Lower Latissmus and Lumbar Rotator Stretch

Sit on the Backbridge and spread your legs in a "V" position. Facing forward, bend your torso over to the right. Bend your right arm and place your right hand on your right hip. Rotate your torso and head to face down, so that you are looking at your right knee. Raise your left arm over your head and straighten it with the palm down, parallel to the floor. Repeat on the opposite side.

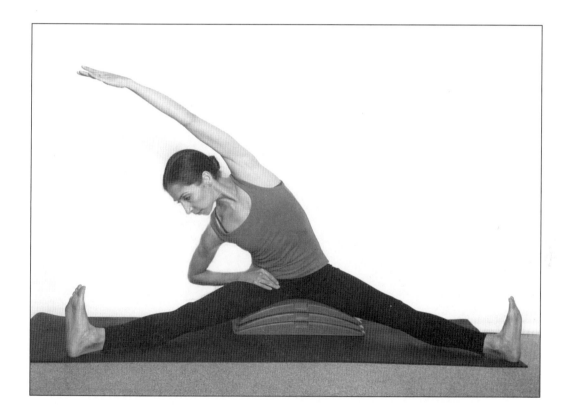

10. Seated Forward Fold

Sitting on the Backbridge as pictured, extend your legs out straight in front of you. Sit tall and fold at the hips, slowly bending forward over your legs as you reach towards your feet. Keep your spine straight and lengthened.

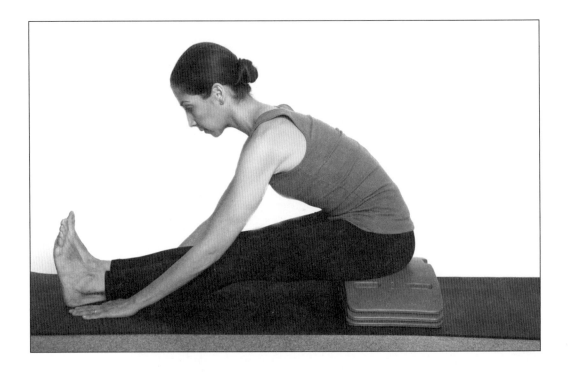

3

Target Your Tight Spots!

In-Depth Stretching for Every Part of Your Body

Got tight hammies? A stiff neck? Tired arms? All your key body parts are listed in this section, with area-specific stretches to help relieve pain and soreness wherever you may have it. While you should regularly do a full body stretch for overall health and flexibility, it's smart to spend a few extra minutes targeting specific overused muscles that are prone to tightness in order to prevent injury and keep you feeling good between longer stretch sessions. These pages are great to turn to when you feel a particular muscle flair up during a run, a tennis game, or just after a long day of sitting at the office.

Remember, the parts of the body are interconnected, and while spot treatments can be helpful, it's also great to do the entire routine when your whole body is feeling in need of a deeper, longer stretch.

LOWER EXTREMITY STRETCHES

ANKLE

Ankle stretches are vital to preventing injuries, especially ankle sprains. Ankle sprains are one of the most common injuries—not just in sports, but for the general public as well. These stretches will improve the range of motion in your ankles and greatly improve something called proprioception, or your body's ability to give you feedback about where it is in space. Improved proprioception will allow for greater athletic performance, fewer injuries and fewer falls. As you stretch the ankle, you might think of moving your foot and ankle as if around the face of a clock. This will optimize stretching by targeting various muscles in the foot, ankle, and shin.

Front Ankle Stretch

Place levels 1 or 2 of the Backbridge on that mat. One foot will be flat on the mat while the top of the other foot will press into the Backbridge. Gently lean into the stretch. Repeat with the opposite foot.

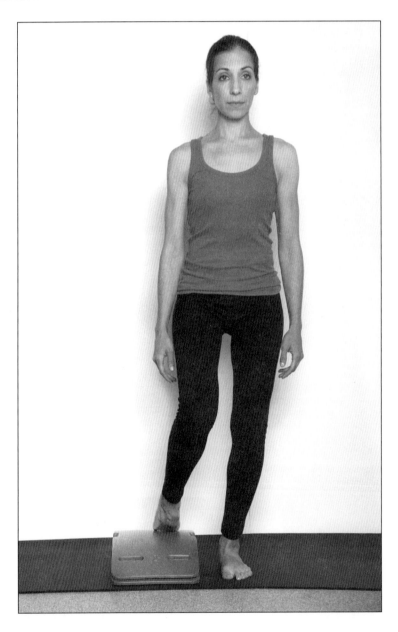

Ankle Eversion

Now, step one foot to the side of the Backbridge, putting the inside of your opposite foot on top of the Backbridge. Place your weight on your standing leg and lean away from the Backbridge, increasing the stretch on the ankle. Repeat with the opposite foot.

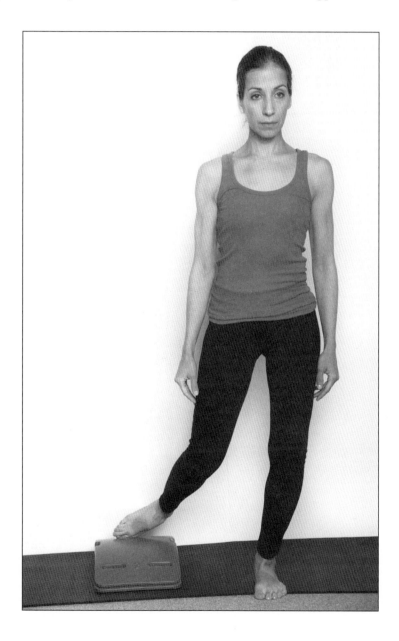

Ankle Inversion

Invert your right ankle, placing the outside of your right foot (pinky toe side) on the Backbridge. Gently press into your right foot. Repeat with the opposite foot.

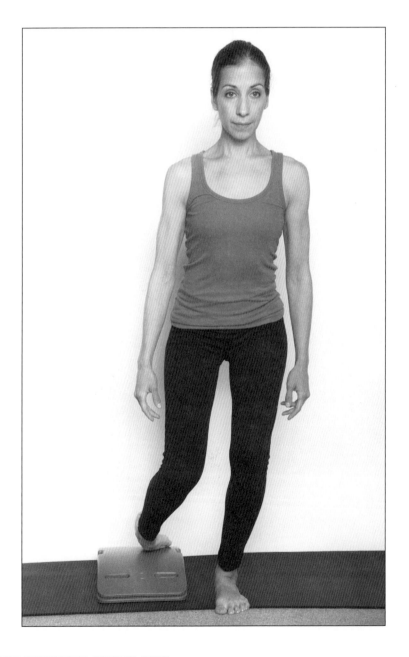

Tibialis Anterior Stretch

This will stretch the ankle as well as the Tibialis Anterior, which runs up the front of your lower leg. A tight Tibialis Anterior is the common cause of shin splints. Place one foot flat on the mat. Place the toes of your other foot face down on the Backbridge and rotate your ankle towards your body so that your toes and ankle are not in a straight line. Lean in so that you feel the stretch in your lower leg. Repeat with the opposite foot.

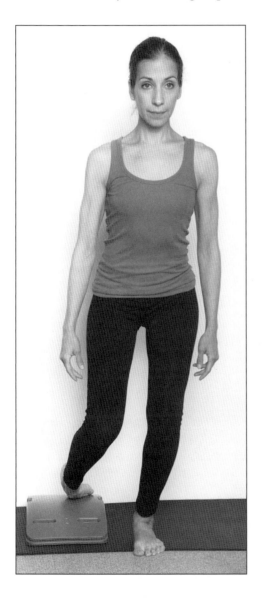
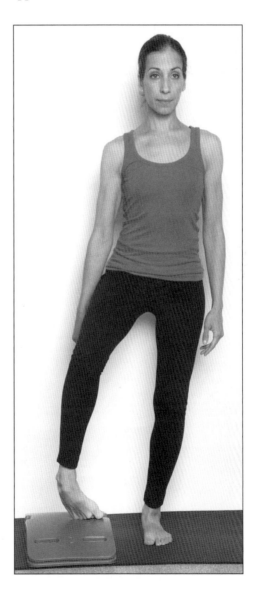

Ankle Stretch Leaning Back

Kneel on the mat and sit back on your heels with the tops of your feet on the Backbridge. Lean back placing your fingertips on the mat beside the Backbridge. This will stretch the Tibialis Anterior or the front part of your ankle and shin.

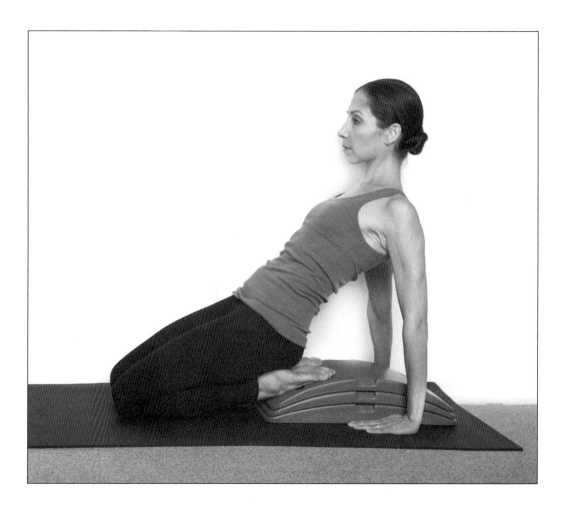

CALF (GASTROCNEMIUS / SOLEUS) AND ACHILLES

The calf muscle, on the back of the lower leg, is actually made up of two muscles:

- ▶ The gastrocnemius is the larger calf muscle, forming the bulge visible beneath the skin. The gastrocnemius has two parts or "heads," which together create its diamond shape.

- ▶ The soleus is a smaller, flat muscle that lies underneath the gastrocnemius muscle.

The gastrocnemius and soleus muscles taper and merge at the base of the calf. Tough connective tissue at the bottom of the calf muscle merges with the Achilles tendon, which inserts into the heel bone (calcaneus). During walking, running, or jumping, the calf muscles pull the heel up to allow forward movement. Calf injuries have become quite common and can be caused by frequently wearing improper shoes which cause undue pressure on the calves. Imbalances in the hips and pelvis also alter our normal walking mechanism and can lead to calf pain.

Calf Stretch with Strap

Sit on the Backbridge at level 2 or 3 and place one leg out straight. Bend your other knee and cross your shin in front of the Backbridge, with the sole of your foot facing the inner thigh of your outstretched leg. Place the strap around your extended foot and gently pull the strap towards you, making sure you sit up straight with a long spine. You should feel the stretch in the calf of your extended leg as well as your ankle and Achilles tendon. Repeat with the opposite leg.

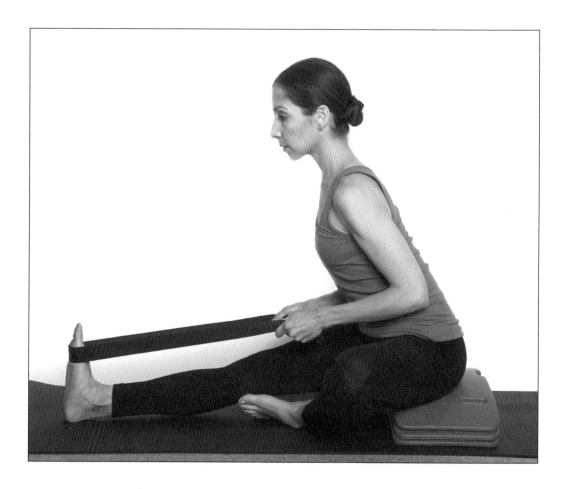

Standing Calf Stretch (Straight Leg)

Using level 2 of the the Backbridge, place your heels on the mat and your toes on the end of the Backbridge.

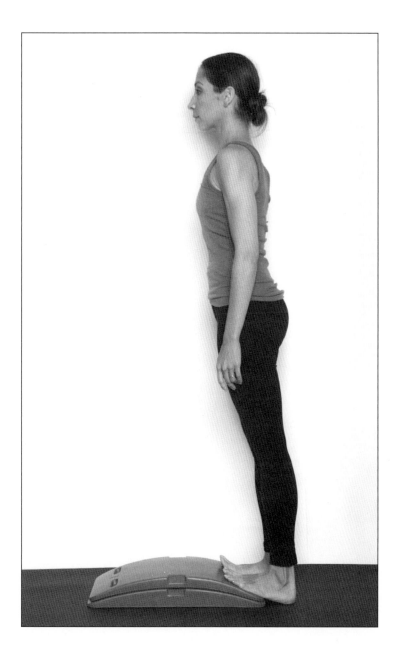

Standing Calf Stretch (Knees Bent)

Using the same form as the previous stretch, gently bend your knees to stretch the upper part of the calf, the soleus muscle.

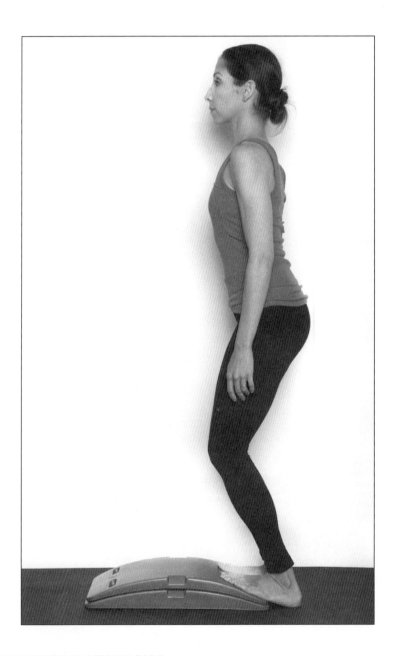

Standing Calf Stretch (on the Backbridge)

Place your toes and the middle of both feet on top of the Backbridge and let your heels hang off the side, reaching toward the mat. Lean forward slightly, shifting your weight over your toes.

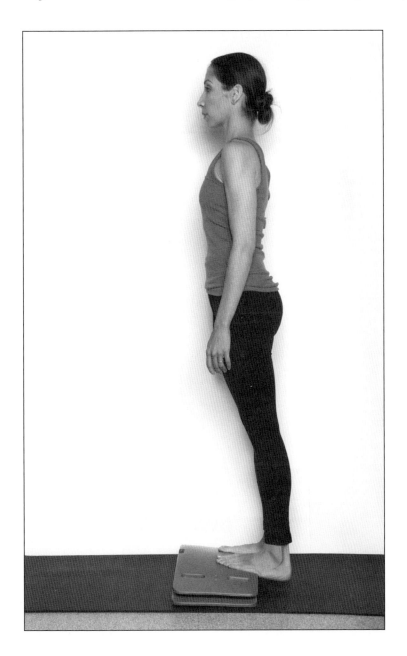

Calf Stretch (Single Leg)

Still standing on the side of the Backbridge, lower down one heel toward the mat, stretching that calf while your other foot remains flat on top of the Backbridge. Repeat with the opposite leg.

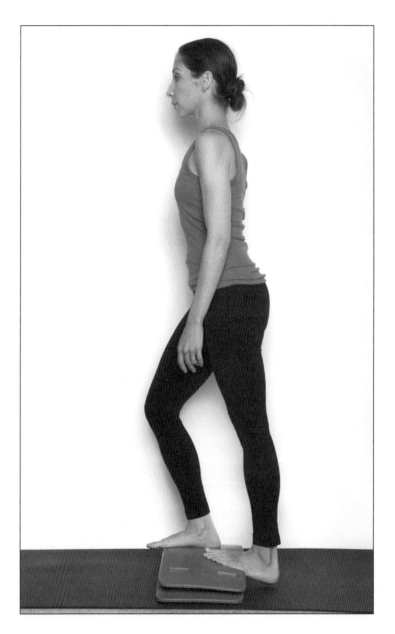

QUADRICEPS

Your quadriceps is the muscle group in the front of your legs between your knees and hips, more commonly known as your thighs. This muscle group helps flex the hips and is vital in lifting, bending, straightening, walking, and running. The quadriceps is the second strongest muscle in the body and is made up of four parts: two muscles (rectus femoris and vastus intermedialis) that pull the knee cap forward, one muscle (vastus lateralis) that pulls it out to the side, and one muscle (vastus medialis) that pulls it towards the midline. All four muscles need to be firing evenly for proper quadriceps and knee function. Imbalances in the quadriceps are frequent causes of knee and hip pain, so stretching is important in maintaining the health and function of this muscle group.

Quadriceps Stretch

Place the front of your left thigh just above the knee on the Backbridge and bring your right leg forward in a lunge position (keeping the knee bent at a 90 degree angle.) Bending your left knee to bring your foot closer to your buttocks, reach back with your left hand and hold your ankle or the top of your foot, slowly leaning forward. The higher the level of the Backbridge you use, the greater the stretch you will feel. Repeat with the opposite leg.

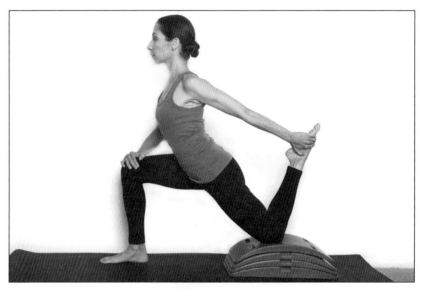

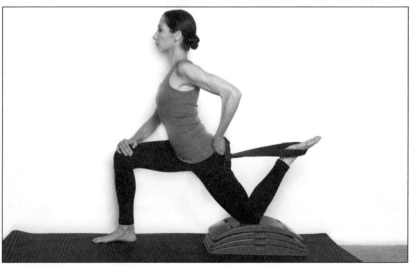

Quadriceps Stretch (Internal and External Rotation)

Stay in your quadriceps stretch position and now slightly pull your ankle towards your midline to work the vastus lateralis muscle (the outer part of your quadriceps), and then gently pull your ankle away from your midline to stretch the vastus medialis muscle (the inner muscle). The model below is showing variations of the stretch with front hand on the floor to increase the stretch and opposite hand grip to change the angle of the stretch. Repeat with the opposite leg.

***If you have knee troubles this stretch could place some undue pressure on your knees, so please be mindful and move with caution.

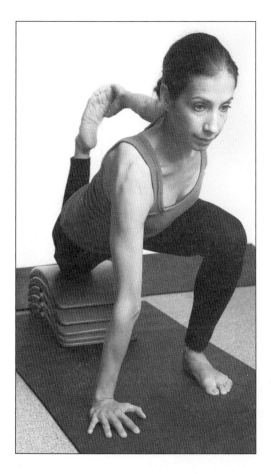
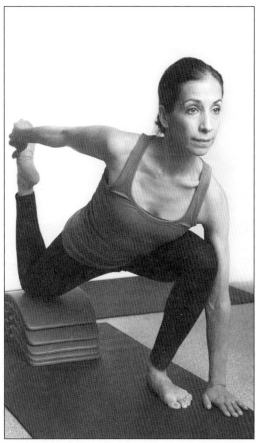

Quadriceps Stretch (Kneeling Position)

Start in the same position as the quadriceps stretch and then lower your front leg to the floor so that your shin and the top of your foot are resting on the mat. Lean forward and rest on your forearm. You can try with the back foot pointed or flexed to change the stretch. Repeat with the opposite leg.

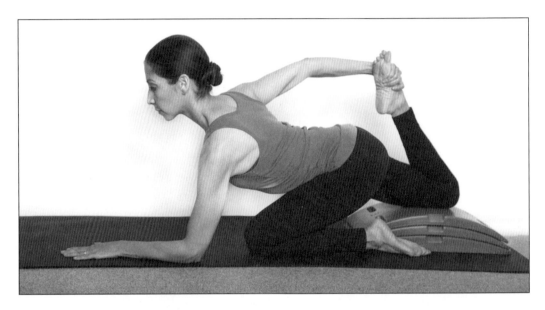

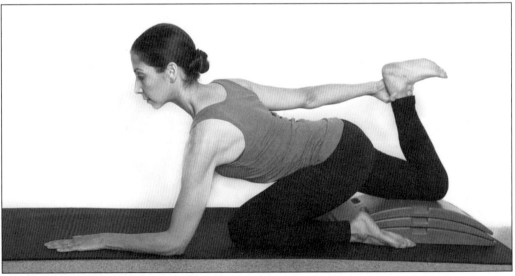

Frog

Place levels 1 and 2 of the Backbridge under one knee and levels 3 and 4 under your other knee. Your knees should be a bit wider than hip width, depending on your flexibility. Bring your feet off the floor and click your heels together in the air behind you. With your body in a modified push up position, lean forward to stretch the front of your quadriceps and hip flexors.

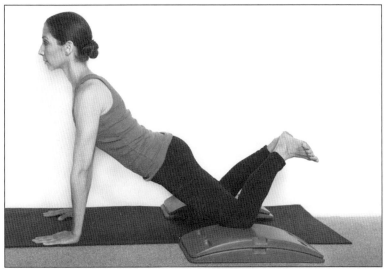

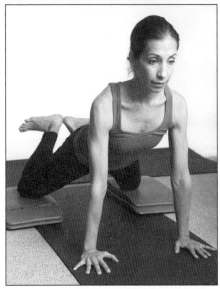

Side-lying heel to buttocks

Lie on your side with your right hip on the highest part of the Backbridge and your right knee bent at a 90 degree angle. You can create a pillow for your head by resting it on your right arm. Bend your left leg and hold on to your left foot with your left hand, gently bringing your heel toward your buttock. This stretch will work not only the quadriceps but also some hip flexors, such as the illiacus and psoas muscles. Repeat on the opposite side.

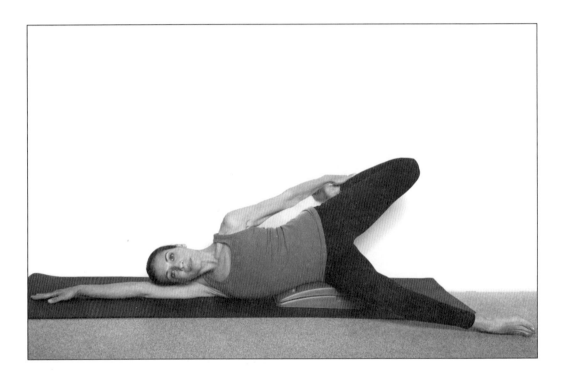

HIP FLEXORS

The hip flexors are a group of skeletal muscles that act to flex the femur (thigh bone) onto the lumbo-pelvic complex, so that you can perform motions like pulling your knee upward.

The hip flexors are composed of two parts:

1. The group collectively known as the iliopsoas or inner hip muscles (in descending order of importance to the action of flexing the hip joint):
   - Psoas major
   - Psoas minor
   - Iliacus muscle

2. The anterior compartment of the thigh, made up of:
   - Rectus femoris (part of the quadriceps muscle group)
   - Sartorius

When the hip flexors get tight, they pull on the pelvis, creating pelvic and hip instability, which results in knee, hip and lower back pain.

Illiopsoas and Illiacus Stretch

Straighten one leg over the Backbridge so that the kneecap rests on the highest point and the top of your foot touches the mat. Position the other leg in front of the Backbridge, bending your knee at a 90 degree angle in a lunge position. With your hands on the mat on either side of your forward foot, lean your body weight forward to stretch the hip flexors in the front of the back leg.

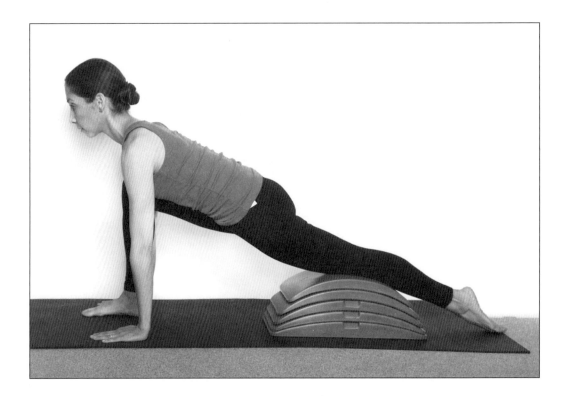

Lunging Hip Flexor Stretch

From the last stretch, lift your torso up and raise your arm opposite your bent knee above your head. Arch back, looking towards the ceiling. Maintain the action of reaching your tailbone to the mat to avoid crunching in the low back. Repeat both stretches on the opposite side.

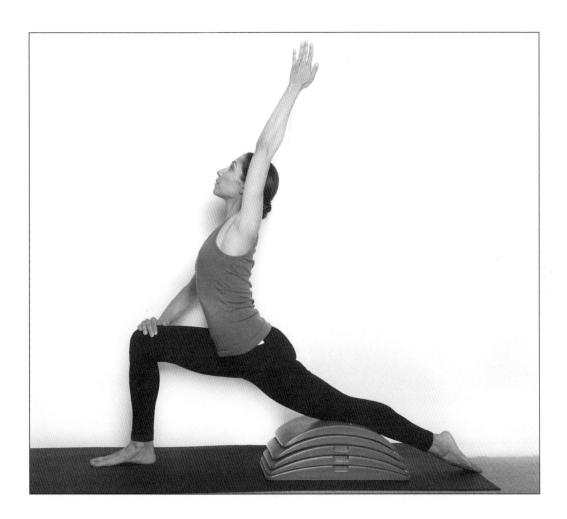

Hip Flexor and Piriformis Stretch (Pigeon Pose)

Using level 1, 2 or 3 of the Backbridge (level 3 giving you the deepest stretch), place one leg, below the knee, on the Backbridge keeping it extended straight behind you. Bend the opposite knee beneath you in front of the Backbridge. The closer the shin is to parallel with the front of the mat, the more intensely you will feel this stretch. There are three different variations of this stretch: 1. sitting up tall, 2. leaning forward onto your forearms, and 3. lying forward with your arms stretched out. Try the different modifications to see which variation works best for you, or use all three. You can also move the Backbridge closer to you, placing it under the buttocks and thigh of your forward, bent leg (as pictured in the second series below). The higher the level of the Backbridge in this position, the easier the stretch will be. Repeat on the opposite side.

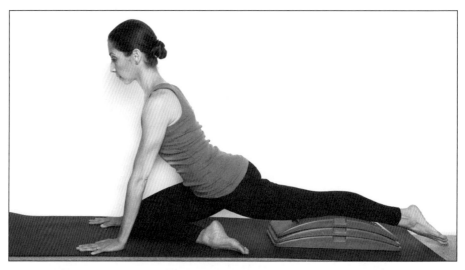

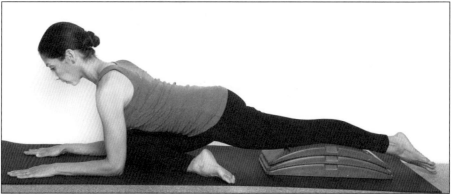

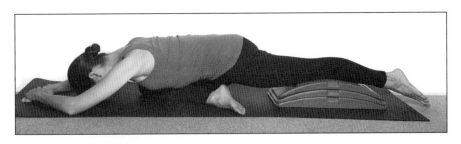

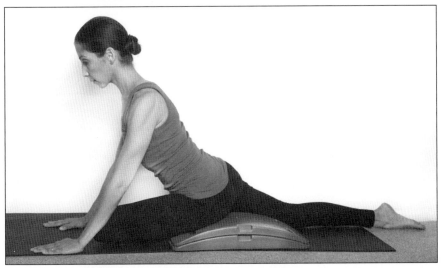

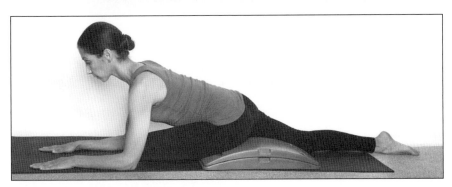

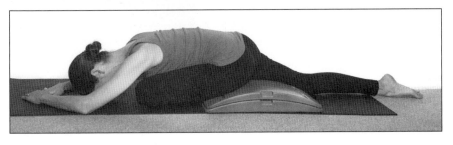

Frog

Place levels 1 and 2 of the Backbridge under one knee and levels 3 and 4 under your other knee. Your knees should be a bit wider than hip width, depending on your flexibility. Bring your feet off the floor and click your heels together in the air behind you. With your body in a modified push up position, lean forward to stretch the front of your quadriceps and hip flexors.

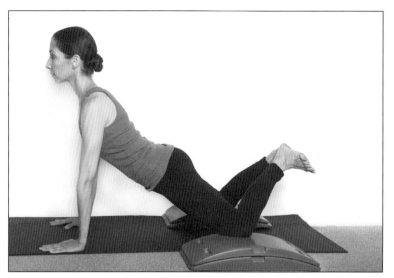

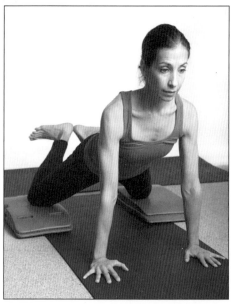

TESNSOR FASCIA LATA AND ILIOTIBIAL BAND

The tesnsor fascia lata (TFL) and the iliotibial band (IT band) form the next muscle group. You can locate these muscles by putting your hands on your hips and feeling the muscle a little to the outside of the bony part of your hip. This is where the TFL attaches. The TFL is only inches long, and it attaches to the IT band, which continues down the outside of your leg and connects below the knee (the IT band also attaches to the gluteus maximus.) These muscles help you lift your leg to the side (hip abduction) and turn your leg inward (internal rotation). They also work to stabilize your hips, pelvis and knees.

Why are these muscles important? Most of the spotlight is usually on the IT band, which is not actually a muscle. It's a thick, dense type of tissue called fascia that connects the TFL to the knee. The IT band gets a lot of attention because it can be a big cause of injury and misalignment of the body if it becomes tight. Knee pain is a particularly common result of a tight TFL & IT band. This is especially true in runners who get what's called IT band friction syndrome. Problems can also arise in the hip and low back because of alignment issues that are caused when the TFL and IT band become tight.

Side-Lying TFL and IT Band Stretch

Lie on your side and place your bottom thigh on top of the Backbridge with your leg extended straight. Bring your top leg across your body and put your foot flat on the floor. Lean your body weight down towards the floor and onto your bottom leg that is on the Backbridge. The higher the level of the Backbridge, the deeper the stretch will be. Repeat on the opposite side.

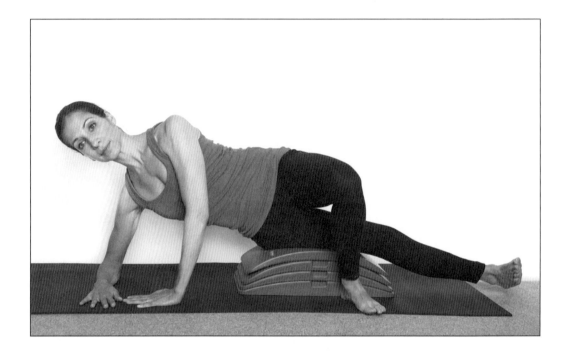

Side-Lying TFL and IT Band (Modified)

Lying on your side with your bottom hip on the highest point of the Backbridge, extend your upper leg straight out. Hook the foot of your lower leg around the calf or ankle of your upper leg so that your bottom knee is slightly bent. With the toes of your hooked foot, apply some downward pressure on your top leg, increasing the amount of stretch on the TFL and IT band. Repeat on the opposite side.

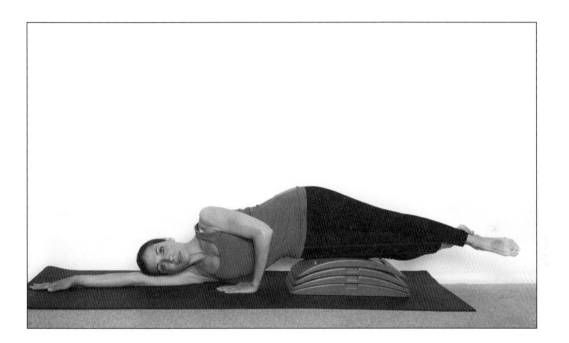

Side-lying TFL and IT Band Stretch (Bent Knee)

Lie on your side just like in the previous stretch, but now bend your top leg slightly, bringing your foot towards your buttocks. Cross your lower leg over your top leg, so that your foot rests on the thigh of your upper leg, just above the knee. With your lower leg, gently apply downward pressure onto your upper leg. The higher the level of the Backbridge, the deeper the stretch will be. Repeat on the opposite side.

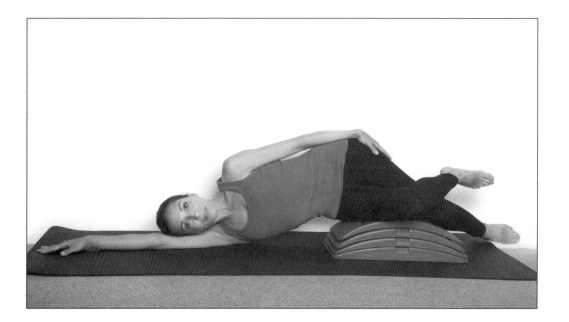

IT Band, TFL, QL and Piriformis Stretch

Lie on your back and twist your leg so your hip is on the highest point of the Backbridge. With bent knees, interlock your upper and lower leg (crossing your top leg over the lower leg with the foot of the top leg hooked on the ankle of the lower leg). Your upper torso and shoulders should remain flat on the mat with your arms extended out in a "T". Repeat on the opposite side.

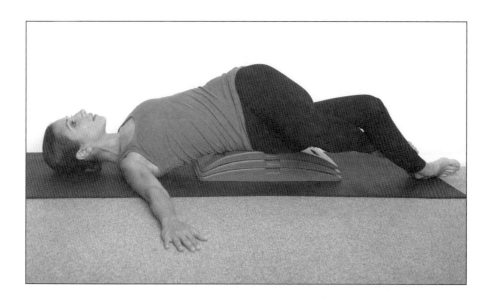

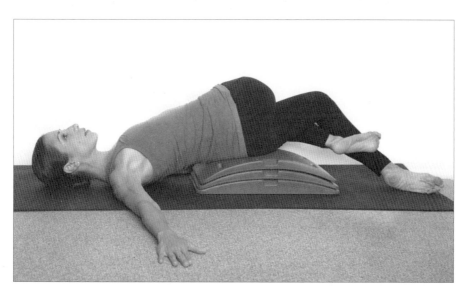

IT Band Stretch (With Strap)

Sit on the highest point of the Backbridge and lie back on the mat. Bring one leg toward your chest and place the stretch strap around your foot just below the ball of your big toe, making sure the strap is flat. Extend your leg straight up above your hip, keeping the other leg extended over the Backbridge or bent with foot on the mat. Gently pull the stretch strap across your body. You should feel this stretch through your hip and along the outside of your thigh. Keep your leg and knee as straight as possible without locking your knee (hyperextension) while doing this stretch. The higher the level of the Backbridge you use, the greater the stretch will be. Repeat on the opposite side.

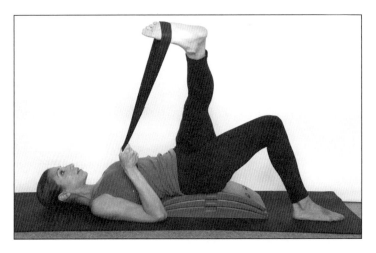

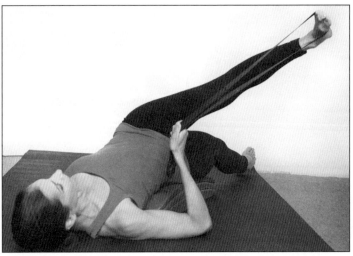

HAMSTRING

The hamstring is involved in knee flexion, hip extension and hyperextension, and transfers power between the hip and knee joints. The biceps femoris, semitendinosus, and semimembranosus are the three muscles that make up the hamstring, located on the back of the leg between the knee and buttocks. When any one of the muscles within this group becomes strained, all three muscles are affected. Hamstring injuries usually occur while engaging in dynamic movements, like running or kicking. Stretching is essential to injury prevention.

Standing Hamstring Stretch

Place one heel on the Backbridge with your other foot flat on the floor. Bend at the waist and attempt to put your whole foot on the Backbridge. Note: the higher the level of the Backbridge, the easier the stretch. Repeat with your other leg. You can also do this stretch with your foot flexed.

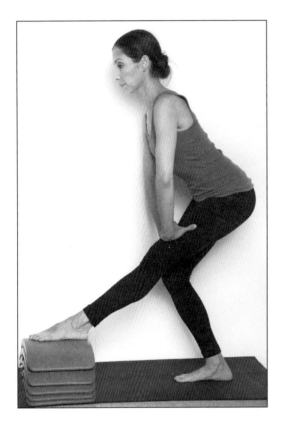
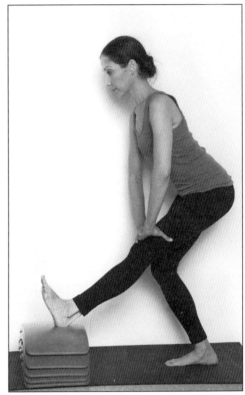

Hamstring Stretch (With Strap)

Sit on the highest point of the Backbridge and lie back on the mat. Bring one leg toward your chest and place the stretch strap around your foot just below the ball of your big toe, making sure the strap is flat. Extend the leg straight up above your hip, keeping the other leg extended over the Backbridge and along the mat. You can modify by bending your other leg and putting your foot on the mat. Gently pull the strap down and back towards your chest to increase the stretch in your hamstring. Keep your leg and knee as straight as possible without locking your knee (hyperextension) while doing this stretch. The higher the level of the Backbridge you use, the greater the stretch will be. Repeat with the other leg.

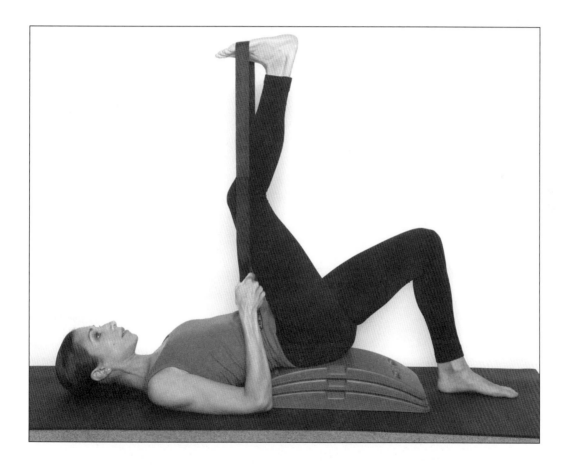

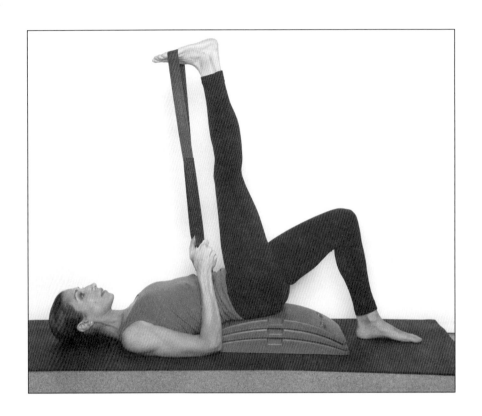

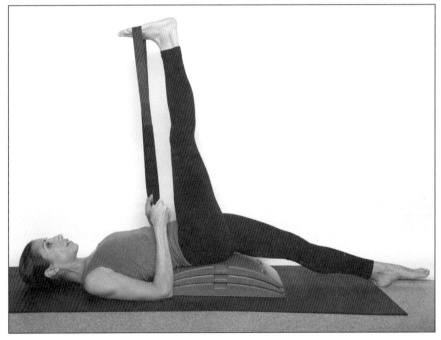

Calf/Hamstring Stretch (With Strap)

Sit on the Backbridge level 2 or 3 and place one leg out straight. Bend your other knee and cross your shin in front of the Backbridge with the sole of your foot facing the inner thigh of your outstretched leg. Place the strap around your extended foot and gently pull the strap towards you, making sure you sit up straight with a long spine. You should feel the stretch in the hamstring of your extended leg, as well as in your calf, ankle and Achilles tendon. Repeat with the other leg.

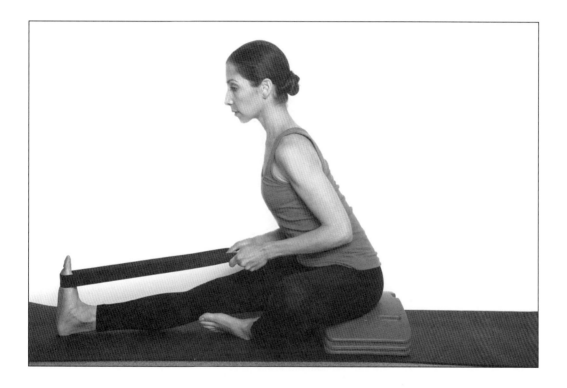

Hamstring and Lower Back Stretch

From the last stretch, bend at the hips and lean forward with a straight back, reaching for the ankle of your outstretched leg. Altering the height of the Backbridge will not necessarily alter the intensity of the stretch, but it will impact different parts of your hamstring, so try different levels to find the stretch you need/prefer. Repeat on the opposite side.

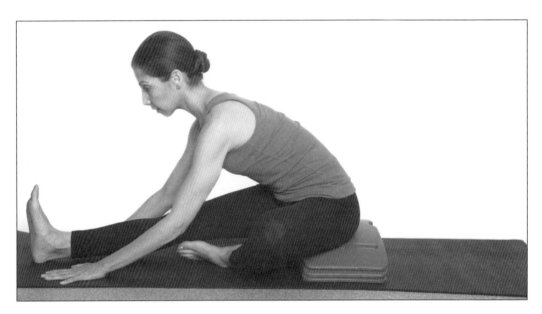

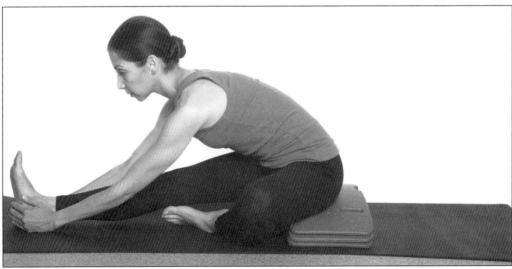

Hamstring and Lower Back Stretch (variation)

From the last stretch, bring your bent leg underneath you with the top of your foot on the mat. the Backbridge will allow you to comfortably sit and stretch in this position without hurting your bent knee. With a straight back, bend at the hip and lean forward reaching for the ankle of your outstretched leg. If you have tight hamstrings, this can also be done with the stretch strap. Repeat on the opposite side.

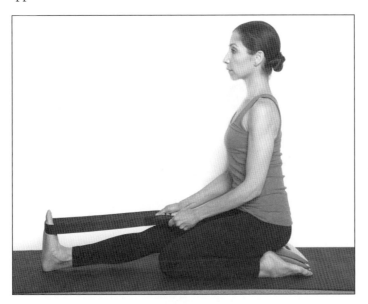

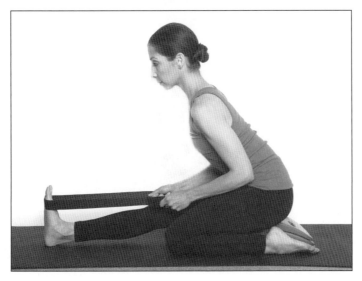

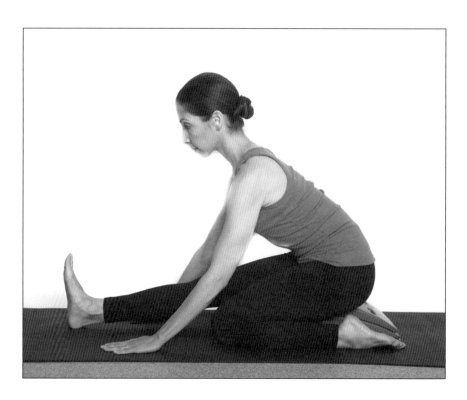

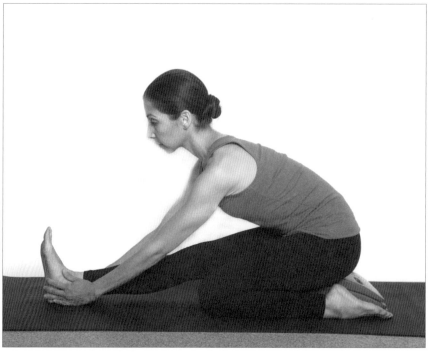

Seated Forward Fold

Sitting on the Backbridge as pictured, extend legs out straight in front of you. Sit tall and folding at the hips, slowly begin to bend forward over your legs, reaching towards your feet. Add the Backbridge levels to increase the stretch.

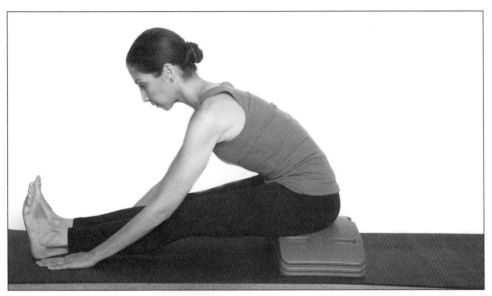

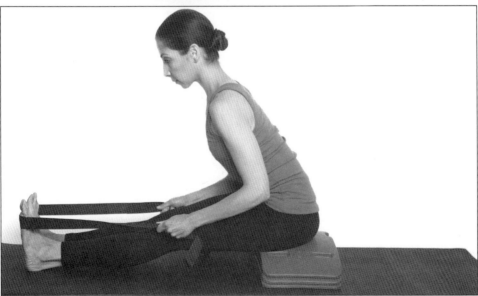

PIRIFORMIS

The piriformis muscle lies directly above your sciatic nerve and impacts your lower back and gluteal muscles. When this muscle is too tight, it can frequently irritate the sciatic nerve and cause piriformis syndrome, a condition characterized by pain, numbness, or a tingling sensation in the buttocks and, sometimes, down the leg. Piriformis syndrome may result from a person's natural anatomy or from overuse or strain of the piriformis muscle. Inactive gluteal muscles and overactive hip flexor muscles can also contribute to the syndrome, as the piriformis muscle becomes overdeveloped in order to compensate. This condition is more common in people who sit down for extended hours, which is the vast majority of the population! A good piriformis stretch can do wonders for your back and hips.

Figure Four Stretch

Sit on the highest point of the Backbridge and lie back on the mat. With one of your legs extended straight up, bend your other leg, crossing your foot over the knee of your extended leg. To avoid strain, be sure that the foot of your bent leg is flexed and extends past, not on top of, the knee of your straight leg. Wrap your hands behind your straight leg and gently pull towards you. Switch legs and repeat.

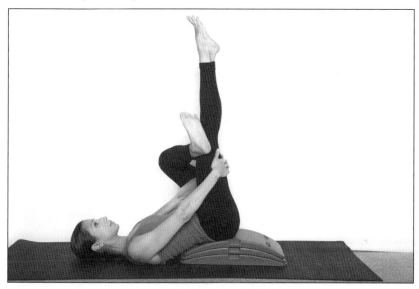

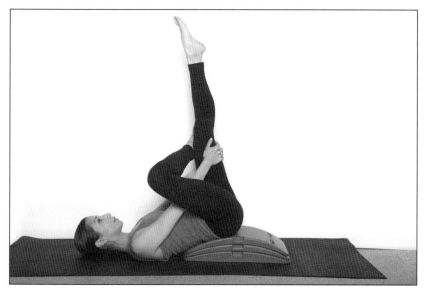

Figure Four (with Legs Bent)

Use the same position as the previous stretch, now bending both of your legs. You will feel this stretch in the back of your leg and buttocks. Switch legs and repeat.

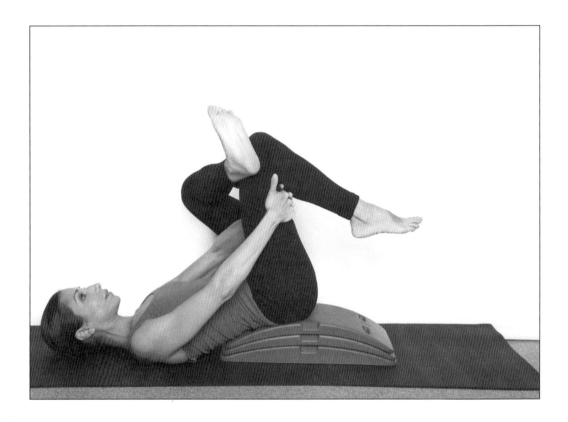

Piriformis Eagle Wrap Twist

Lie on your side with your hip on the highest point of the Backbridge, and with bent knees, interlock your upper and lower leg (crossing your top leg over the lower leg with the foot of the top leg hooked on the ankle of the lower leg). Your upper torso and shoulders should remain flat on the mat with your arms extended out in a "T". Repeat on opposite side.

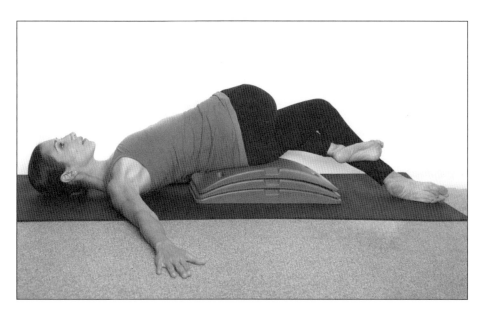

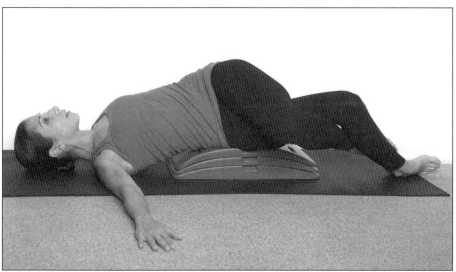

Piriformis Stretch in Pigeon Pose

Using level 1, 2 or 3 of the Backbridge (level 3 giving you the deepest stretch), place one leg, below the knee, on the Backbridge, keeping it extended straight behind you. Bend the opposite knee beneath you in front of the Backbridge. The closer the shin is to parallel with the front of the mat, the more intensely you will feel this stretch. There are three different variations of this stretch: 1) sitting up tall, 2) leaning forward onto your forearms, and 3) lying forward with your arms stretched out. Try the different modifications to see which variation works best for you, or use all three. You can also move the Backbridge closer to you, placing it under the buttocks and thigh of your forward, bent leg (as pictured in the second series below). The higher the level of the Backbridge in this position, the easier the stretch will be. Switch legs and repeat.

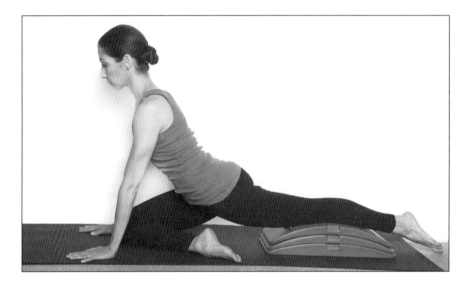

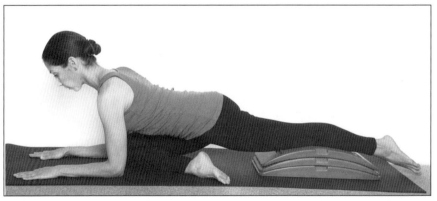

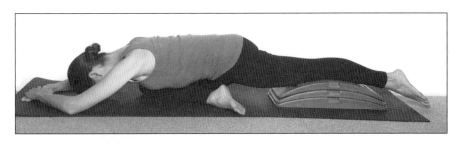

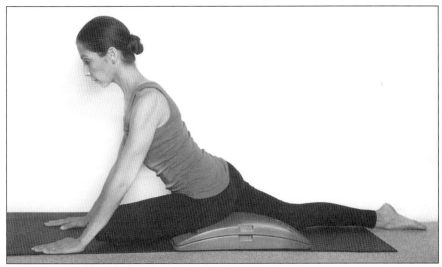

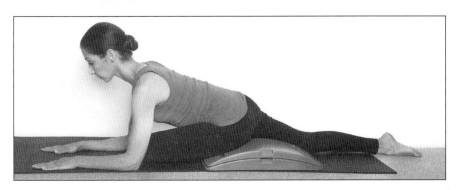

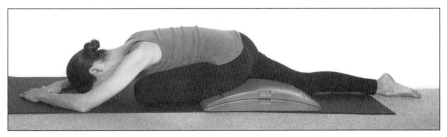

INNER THIGH AND GROIN

The groin muscles are a group of muscles situated high on the leg in the inner thigh. This group includes the adductor magnus, adductor longus, and adductor brevis muscles, as well as the pectineus and gracilis muscles. Collectively referred to as the hip adductors, the groin muscles are responsible for adduction of the hip, or drawing the leg in toward the midline of the body. These muscles can get injured when we move side to side or frequently perform stops and starts in our activity. Inner thigh and groin injuries are particularly predominant in football, soccer and tennis players.

Inner Thigh and Groin Stretch

Sit in a cross-legged position on the Backbridge, placing your ankles in front of one another with the tops of your feet on the mat and your hands on your knees. Feel a gentle opening in your thighs, hips and groin. Hold for 20 seconds, then switch the cross of the ankles.

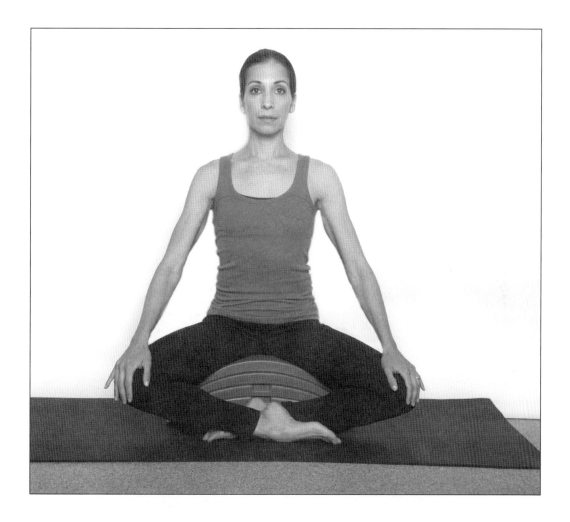

Inner Thigh and Groin Stretch (Butterfly)

Sit on the Backbridge and pull your feet in as close as possible. Place the soles of the feet together, letting the knees slowly drop open towards the mat. You can gently push down on your thighs with your elbows or on your lower legs with your forearms to increase the stretch. Using higher levels of the Backbridge will help people with tight hips by allowing your knees to drop open, similar to sitting on a block or blanket in yoga. As always, listen to your body and find the level that is best for you.

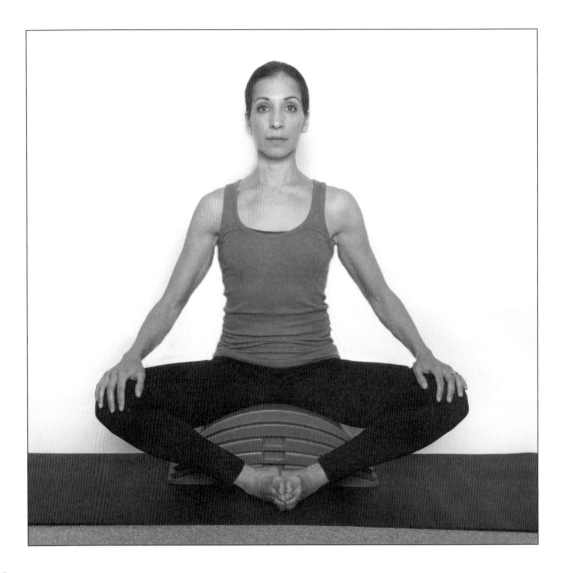

Seated Wide Angle Stretch

Sit on top of the Backbridge with your legs extended straight out to the sides in a wide "V" position. You may point or flex your feet to alter the stretch as well as varying the level of the Backbridge to change the intensity of the stretch (level 5 being the hardest).

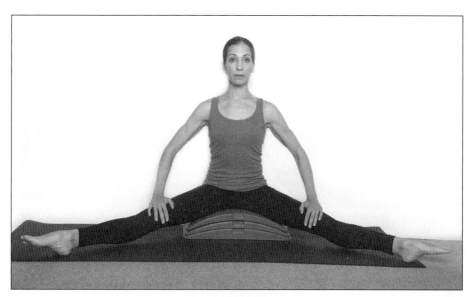

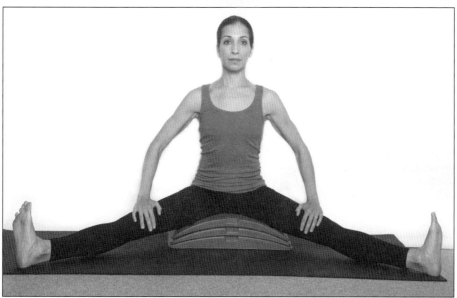

Groin and Inner Thigh Forward Stretch

Sit on the Backbridge with legs spread in a "V." Keeping your back as straight as possible, hinge forward at hips, bringing your forearms to the mat.

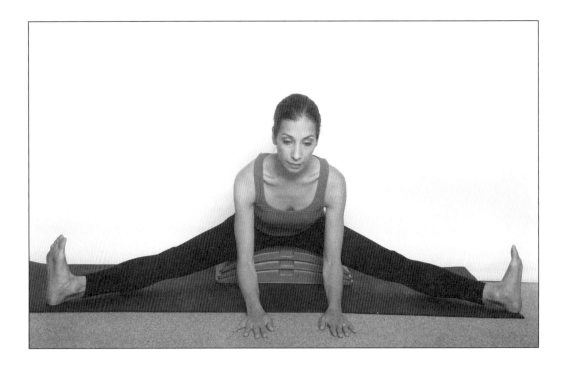

Inner Thigh Lunge

Place one foot on the Backbridge and step wide with your other foot, putting about one leg's distance between your feet. Bend your knee and shift your weight to your outside leg, lunging to the side. Be sure that your knee does not extend beyond your toes. The deeper you go into the lunge, the greater the stretch you will feel. Increasing the level of the Backbridge will also intensify the stretch. Repeat on the opposite side.

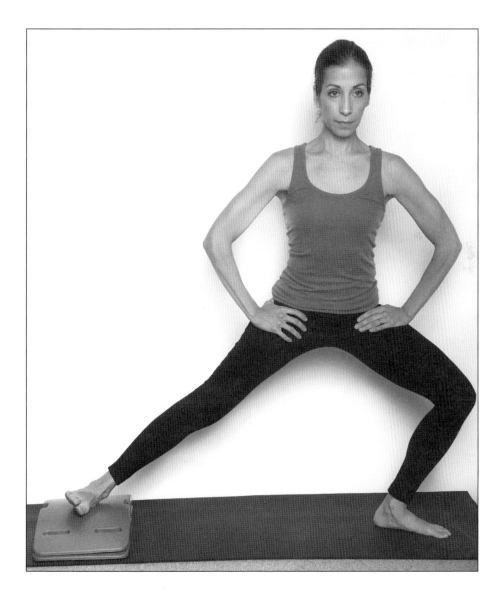

QUADRATUS LUMBORUM

The quadratus lumborum, or QL, connects the pelvis to the spine and is a common source of lower back pain. Constant contraction (habitual seated computer use and/or the use of a lower back support in a chair) can overuse the QLs, resulting in muscle fatigue. A constantly contracted QL, like any other muscle, will experience decreased blood flow, and, in time, adhesions in the muscle and fascia may develop, the end point of which is muscle spasm.

QL Stretch (with Hand Assist)

Lying face up with your buttocks on the highest point of the Backbridge, extend one of your legs out straight on the mat and bend and cross your other leg over it so that your foot rests on the mat. Place your hand on the thigh of your bent leg, gently applying downward pressure. Slowly try to bring your bent knee to the mat. Repeat on the opposite side.

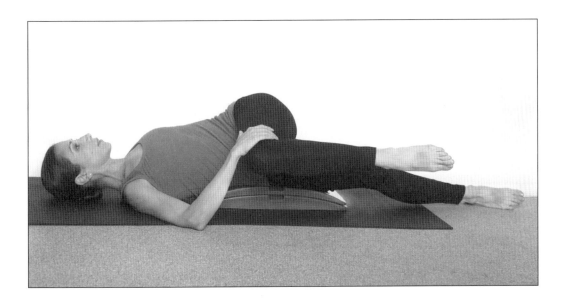

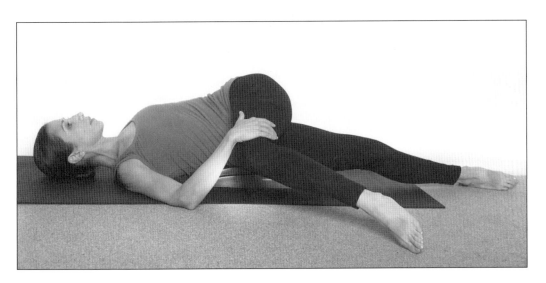

QL Stretch From a Split Position

Sit on the Backbridge and spread your legs in a "V" position. Facing forward, bend your torso over to the right, sliding your right arm down your right leg. Raise your left arm over your head, so that your upper arm is next to your ear. Keep your palm open and facing the floor. Rotate your torso and head slowly towards the ceiling to open the chest, feeling the stretch in your lower back. Repeat on opposite side.

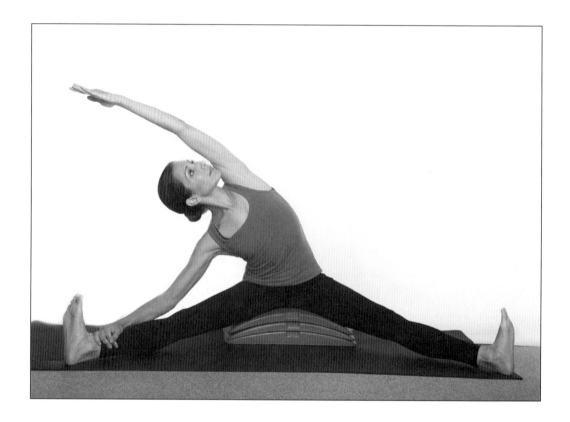

QL Stretch (with Stretch Strap)

Sit on the highest point of the Backbridge and lie back on the mat. Bring one leg toward your chest and place the stretch strap around your foot just below the ball of your big toe, making sure the strap is flat. Extend your leg straight up above your hip, keeping the other leg extended over the Backbridge and along the mat. Gently pull the stretch strap across your body. You should feel this stretch through your hip and along the outside of your thigh. Keep your leg and knee as straight as possible without locking, or hyperextending, your knee while doing this stretch. The higher the level of the Backbridge you use, the greater the stretch will be. Switch legs and repeat.

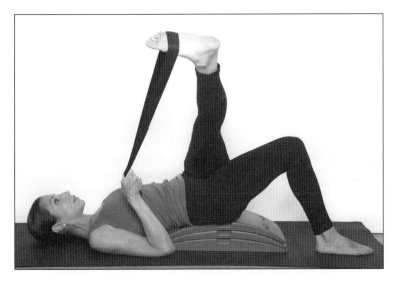

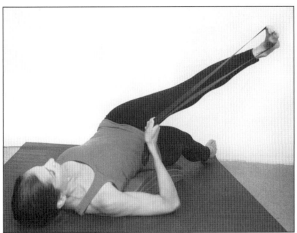

LUMBAR PARASPINAL MUSCLES

The paraspinal muscles are the muscles that run next to, and roughly parallel with, the spine. They consist of many small muscles that are attached to the vertebrae and control the motion of the individual bones, as well as assist with the larger motions of the whole trunk, or core, area. Together with other muscles, they help support the spine and keep it in proper vertical alignment. They also limit the range of motion of the spine, which helps to prevent injuries to the discs and spinal cord caused by overextension.

In human anatomy, nearly all skeletal muscles work in pairs. While one muscle is contracting, or getting shorter, another muscle must get longer to allow movement. When a person bends forward, his/her paraspinal muscles lengthen; when he/she stands up again, they contract to pull him/her back to a standing position. Paraspinal muscles on the left and right side of the body work together in the same way when a person bends sideways. It is important to keep these muscles limber for proper movement.

Seated Forward Fold

Sitting on the Backbridge as pictured, extend your legs out straight in front of you. Sit tall and fold at the hips, slowly bending forward over your legs, reaching towards your feet. The higher levels of the Backbridge will be helpful for those people with tight hips, but may not allow you to go as deep in the stretch. As always, listen to your body and try different levels to change the stretch and figure out what level works best for you.

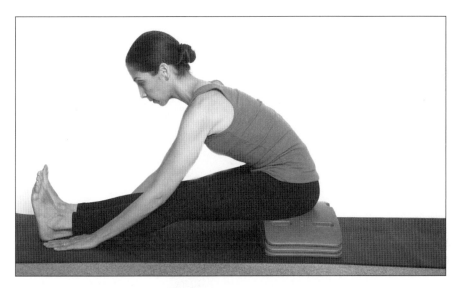

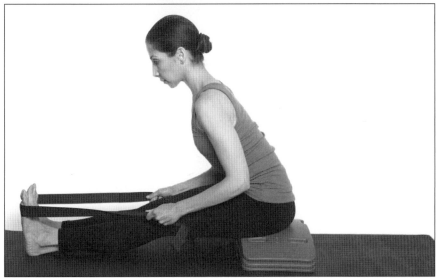

Lower Back Stretch

From the last stretch, bring your bent leg underneath you with the top of your foot on the mat. the Backbridge will allow you to comfortably sit and stretch in this position without hurting your bent knee. With a straight back, bend at the hip and lean forward, reaching for the ankle of your outstretched leg. If you have tight hamstrings, this can also be done with the stretch strap. The higher the level on the Backbridge, the larger the stretch in the hamstrings and the less in lower back. So, the lower levels of the Backbridge will impact you more in the lower back and less in the hamstring. Switch legs and repeat.

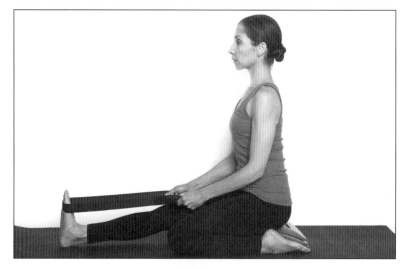

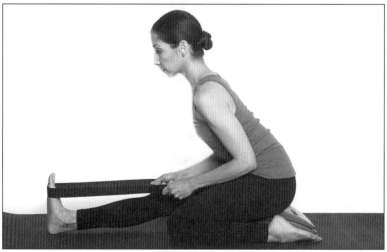

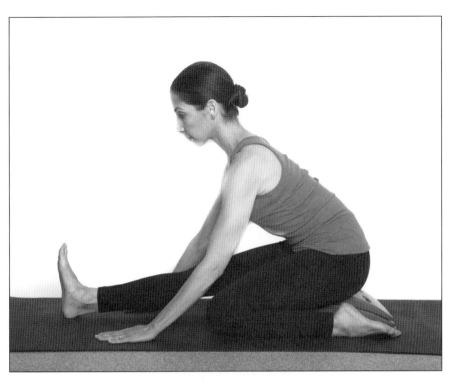

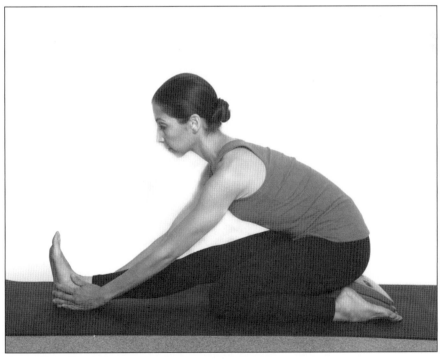

Lower Back Stretch (variation)

From the last stretch, bend one leg and place the sole of the foot to the inner thigh of the outstretched leg. Bend at the hips and lean forward with a straight back, reaching for the ankle of your outstretched leg. Altering the height of the Backbridge will not necessarily alter the intensity of the stretch, but it will impact different muscles, so try different levels to find the stretch you need/prefer. Switch legs and repeat.

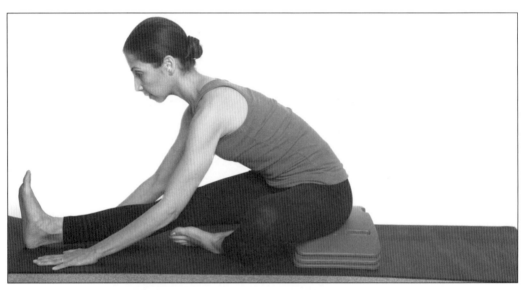

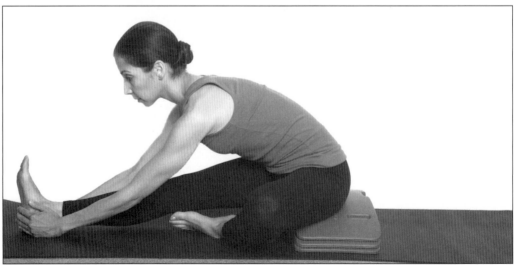

Lumber Paraspinal Stretches From A Split Position

Sit on the Backbridge and spread your legs in a "V" position. Facing forward, bend your torso over to the right, sliding your right arm down your right leg. Raise your left arm over your head, so that your upper arm is next to your ear. Keep your palm open and facing the floor. Rotate your torso and head slowly towards the ceiling to open the chest, feeling the stretch in your lower back. Repeat on opposite side.

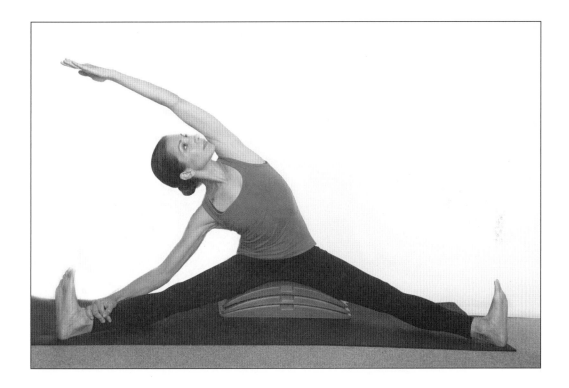

Stay in the last stretch, but now bend your right arm and place your right hand on your right hip. Rotate your torso to face forward and your head to face down, so that you are looking at your right knee. Your left arm should remain straight with your palm down, parallel to floor.

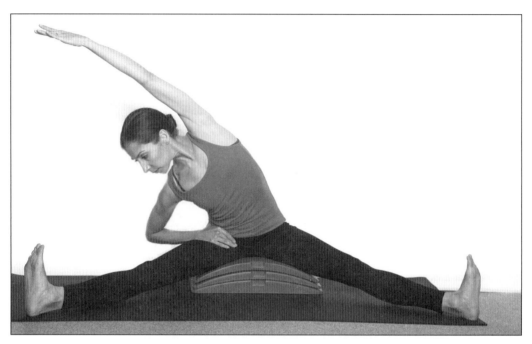

Still sitting in a split position, rotate your torso down and reach for your right foot with both hands.

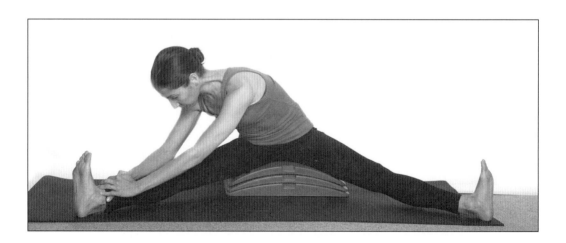

Cobra Stretch

Lie face down over the Backbridge and place your hands in front of you. Do half a push up so that your upper torso is elevated, but your pelvis still has contact with the Backbridge. Look straight ahead and hold for a count of 5, then slowly lower yourself down and repeat. This stretch really works your lumbar extenders and lower back while stretching and lengthening the core (abdominals). The higher the level of the Backbridge you use, the easier the stretch will be.

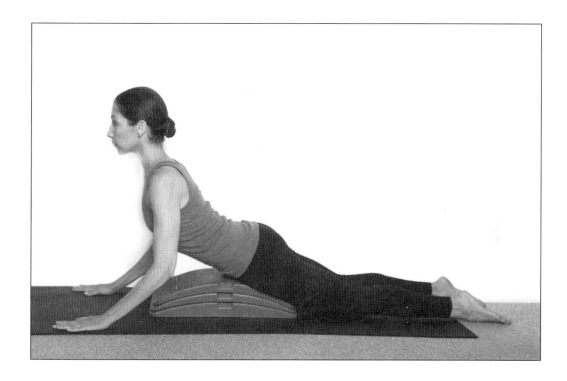

Cobra Stretch (With Head Turn)

Doing the same cobra stretch, turn your head to the side and try to look behind you. This variation will stretch the lower lumbar musculature differently. Look over the opposite shoulder.

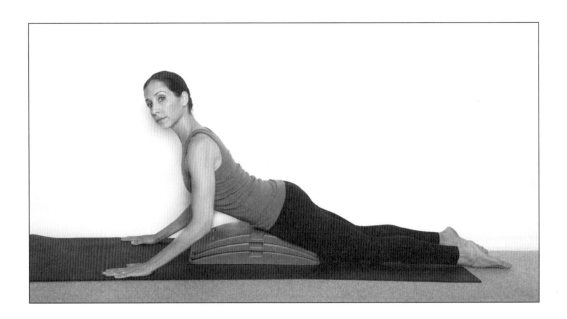

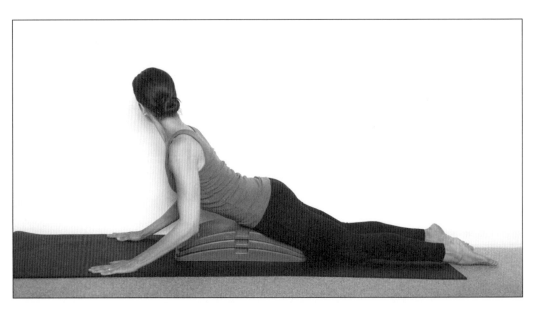

Reclining Twist

Place the Backbridge about 12 inches to the side of your hips. Extend your arms to the side in a "T," keeping your shoulders flat on the mat and bring one knee towards your chest. With your other leg flat on the mat, pull your bent knee over your torso, placing it on the Backbridge. Try different levels of the Backbridge to find which is most comfortable for you (level 1 is the hardest.) If you can comfortably rest on level 1, try bringing your knee to the ground. The key to this stretch is keeping your shoulders on the mat. Repeat on the opposite side.

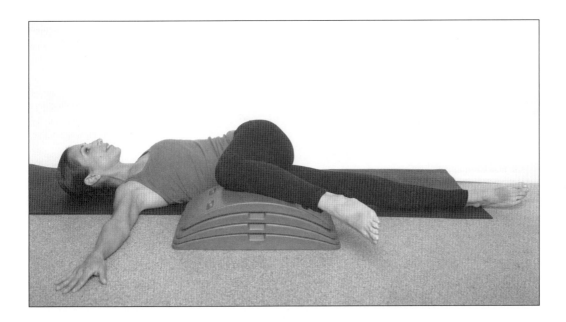

Knees To Chest Stretch

For a low back stretch, place your buttocks on the highest point of the Backbridge and lay back on the mat. Wrap your hands around your knees and gently pull your knees to your chest while reaching and lengthening your tailbone down towards the Backbridge. Hold for a few seconds. If you have trouble wrapping your hands around your knees, you can place them behind your legs on the backs of your thighs. The higher level of the Backbridge you use in this posture, the more intense the stretch.

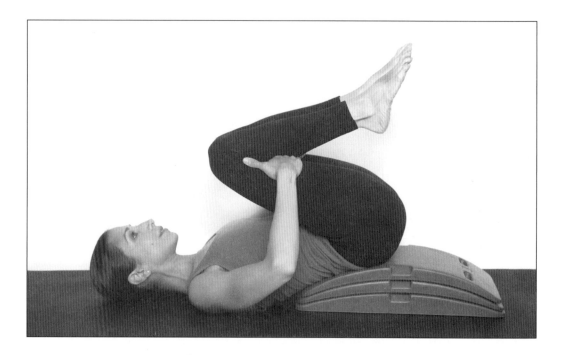

Single Knee To Chest Stretch

Set up like the Knee to Chest stretch, but pull one leg toward your chest and extend the opposite leg over the Backbridge and along the mat. By gently angling the knee inward or outward, you will stretch different parts of your hip flexors. For a less intense stretch, you may also keep the leg bent if it's more comfortable on your low back or hip flexor. Switch legs and repeat.

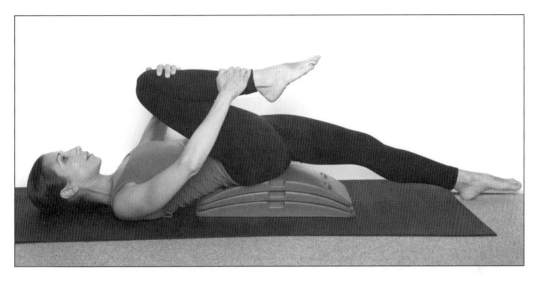

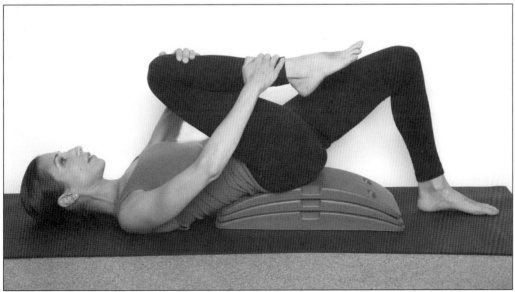

Sacral Stretch

Place the Backbridge perpendicular to your body. Lie back over the Backbridge and position your sacrum (center of low back, between your hips) on the highest point. Bend your knees, placing your feet on the ground. The higher the level of the Backbridge that you use, the greater the stretch you will feel.

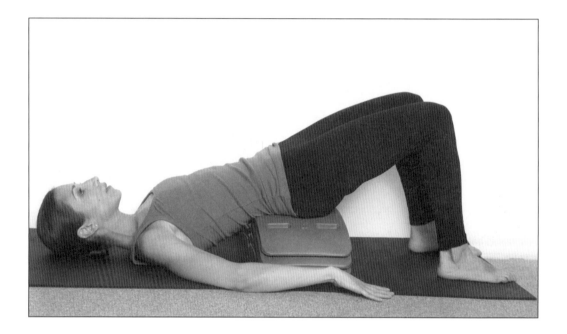

MID AND UPPER BACK

The muscles of the mid to upper back consist of the latissimus dorsi (the lats), the rhomboids and the trapezius (traps). Aside from providing stability to your spine, the upper back muscles are also prominently used during any sort of pulling motion, as in rowing or tug of war.

The lats are a triangular-shaped muscle responsible for adduction (movement **towards** the body), internal rotation and extension of the shoulder joint. The lats are also very important in stabilizing the spine during extension (backward bending) and flexion (forward bending) of the back. Because the lats are also attached to the inside of the upper arm, it's easy to understand that when the muscle shortens, they help rotate the arm inwards and pull the upper arm closer to the body. Any motion that pulls your arms back towards your body, like pull-ups, pull-downs, rowing, or cable crossovers, is working your lats.

Rhomboids are comprised of the rhomboid major and the rhomboid minor. When the rhomboid major shortens, the shoulder blades are pulled together. Extending an already extended shoulder joint is its function. Most people with poor posture also have very weak rhomboids because their back is always supported by a chair.

The traps are diamond-shaped muscles that lie on top of the rhomboids and part of the lats. The basic actions of the traps include retracting the shoulder blades (pulling them together) and both depressing and elevating them (shrugging your shoulders). The traps additionally function to stabilize the shoulder joint and allow you to tilt your head back.

Because injuries occur when the shoulder joint is weak, keeping the traps strong and flexible can help to avoid seemingly unrelated problems, like back and neck pain.

Side Lying Stretch

Lie on your side and stretch over the Backbridge so that the highest point of the Backbridge is at your rib cage. With your bottom hand, grab the wrist of your top hand and extend your arms overhead along the ground. As you progress, add more levels of the Backbridge to increase the stretch. Repeat on the opposite side.

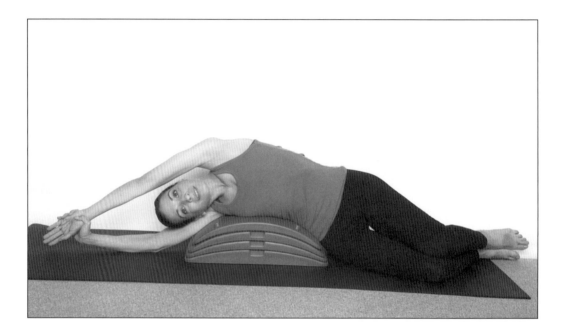

Shoulder and Torso Stretches

Sitting back on your knees, place your forearms on the Backbridge shoulder width apart, with your palms facing each other (thumbs toward the ceiling). Lie forward as much as possible with your head between your upper arms. This will open up both your shoulders and your chest.

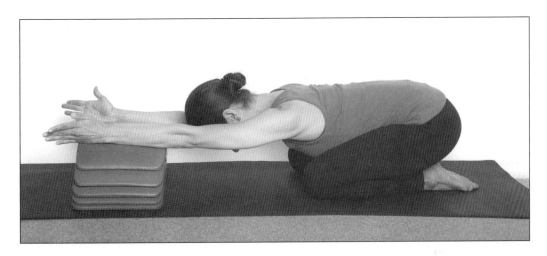

From the last stretch, interlock your fingers and lean back, trying to bring your buttocks to your heels.

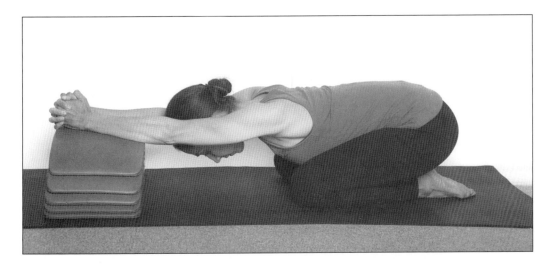

Shoulder and Torso Stretch With Twist

From the last stretch, keep your fingers interlocked and twist your arms so that one hand rolls on top of other. Hold and then repeat on other side, switching the interlock of your hands and twisting in the opposite direction.

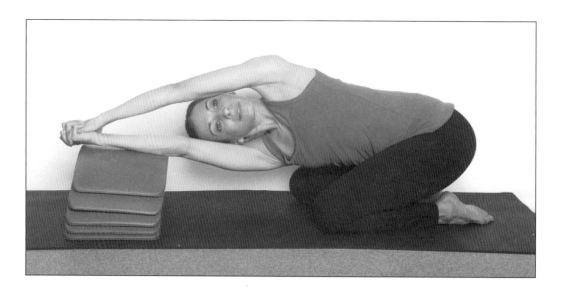

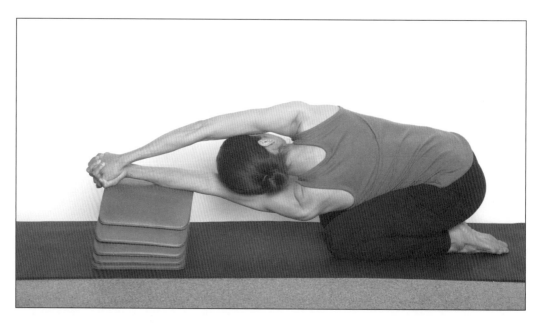

Shoulder Stretch With Intercrossed Arms

Sit back on your knees, straighten your arms, turn them face up, and cross them at the elbows. Lean forward so that your arms rest on the Backbridge and your head rests on your upper arms. Hold and then repeat, re-crossing arms with your opposite arm on top. You can try this same stretch with palms facing down for a slightly different sensation.

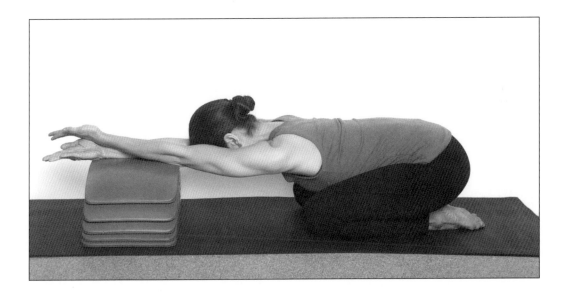

PECTORALIS MAJOR AND MINOR (CHEST MUSCLES)

The Pectoralis muscles (pecs) attach the sternum (breast bone), ribcage, and clavicle (collar bone) to the humerus (upper arm bone). When working with certain muscles of the back (like the lats), the pecs share the function of adducting the arm (pulling it down and in towards the body). When working alone, they pull the arm forward.

Side-Lying Chest Stretch

While side lying on the Backbridge, raise your upper arm and extend it back so that your chest opens to the ceiling. Angle this arm in slightly different directions to stretch various fibers of your pecs. Repeat on the opposite side.

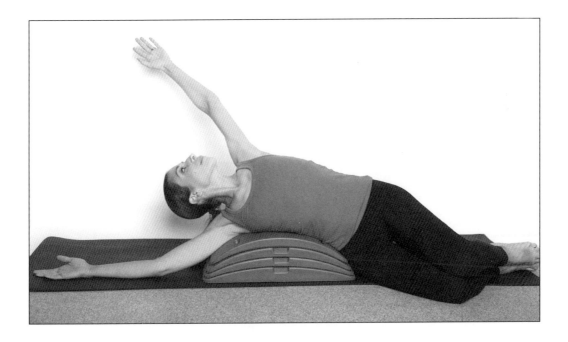

Standing Abdominal Twist

Standing up, place the Backbridge about 10 inches in front of you, perpendicular to your body. Standing with feet about a mat's width apart, bend forward at the hips, keeping a flat back and straight legs. Stretch your arms out into a "T" position and rotate your torso to touch the Backbridge with your fingertips, letting your other arm extend toward the ceiling. Look up in the direction of your raised arm to open your chest further. Rotate your torso to the opposite side.

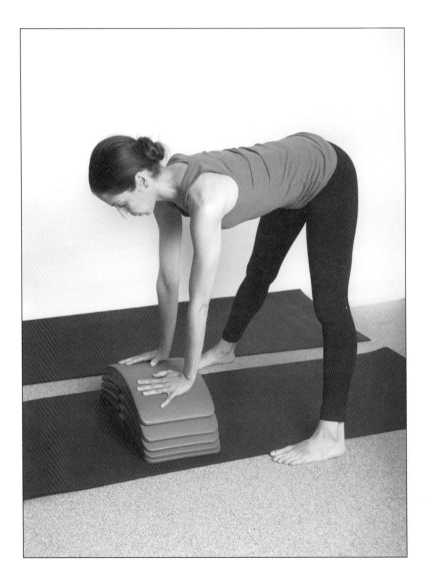

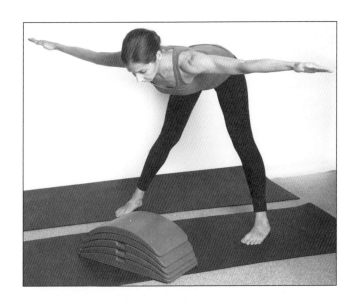

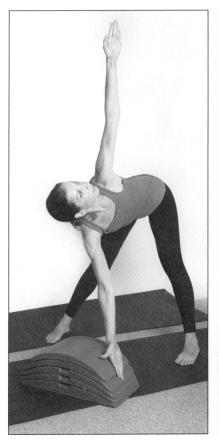

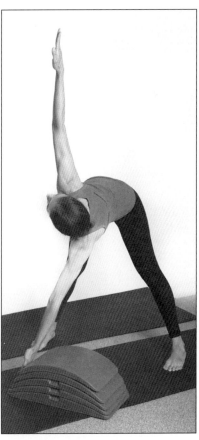

Chest Opener

Set up the Backbridge on level 4 or 5, and sit in front of it so that your lower back is even with the end. Lean back, letting your straight arms drape to sides to open your chest muscles.

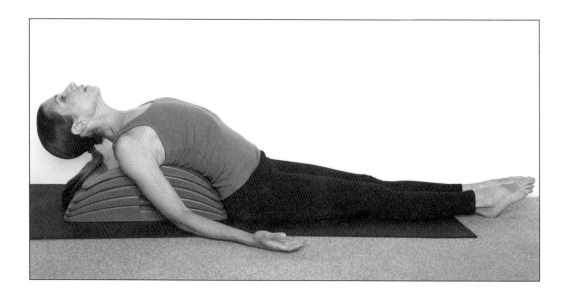

Pectoralis Stretch (Face Down)

Lying face down on the mat, place the Backbridge to your side about a foot from your arm. Put your forearm and elbow on top of the Backbridge, hand facing down with your elbow bent at a 90 degree angle. Increase your the Backbridge level to get a greater stretch. Repeat on the opposite side.

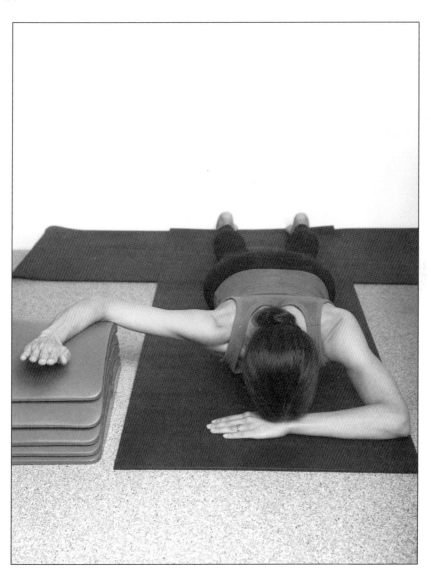

Pectoralis Stretch (Modification)

To modify the previous stretch, turn your head away from the Backbridge and rest it on your opposite arm. Repeat on the opposite side.

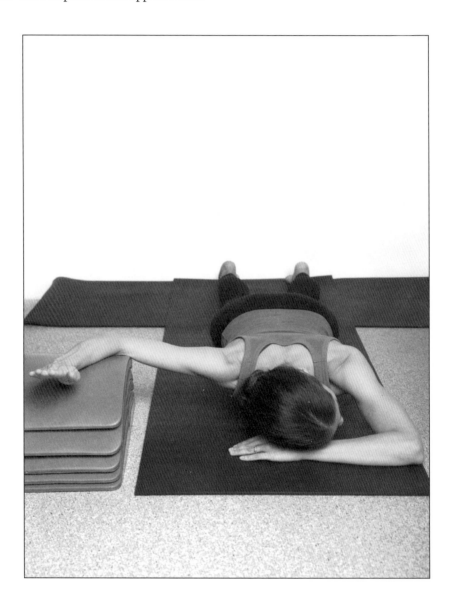

ROTATOR CUFF (SHOULDER MUSCLES)

The rotator cuff is made up of four muscles: the supraspinatus, the infraspinatus, the teres minor, and the subscapularis. Often the mnemonic *SITS* is used to help remember these muscles. These individual muscles combine at the shoulder to form a thick "cuff" over the joint. The rotator cuff has the important job of stabilizing the shoulder, as well as elevating and rotating the arm. Each muscle originates on the shoulder blade, or scapula, and inserts on the upper arm bone, or humerus. The muscles abduct, or elevate, the shoulder joint; stabilize the head of the humerus in the shoulder joint; externally rotate the shoulder joint; and depress the head of the humerus.

Shoulder And Torso Stretch

Sitting on your knees, place your forearms on the Backbridge, interlock your fingers and lie forward as much as possible with your head between your upper arms. Leaning back, try to bring your buttocks to your heels. This will open up your shoulders and chest.

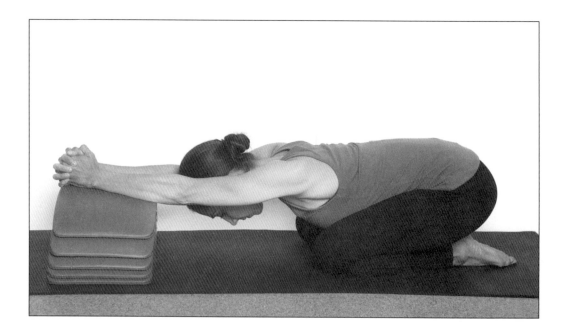

Shoulder and Torso Stretch with Twist

Sitting back on your knees, interlock your hands and lie forward so that your fists rest on the Backbridge. Twist your arms so that one hand rolls on top of other. Hold and then repeat on other side, switching your hands and twisting in the opposite direction.

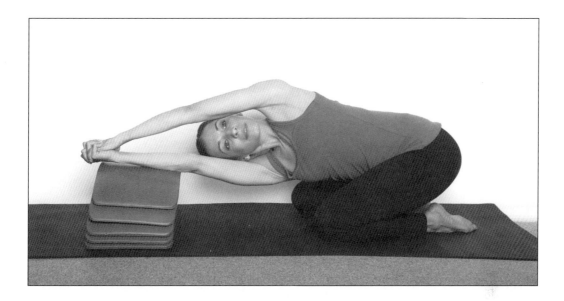

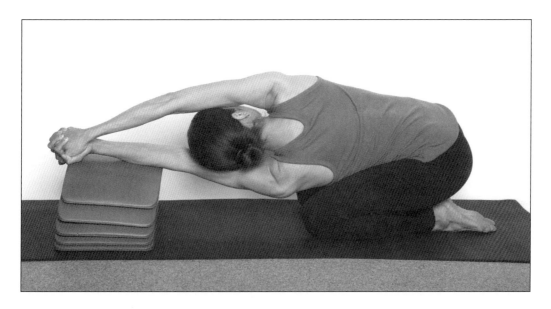

Shoulder Stretch With Intercrossed Arms

Sit back on your knees, straighten your arms, turn them face up, and cross them at the elbows. Lean forward so that your arms rest on the Backbridge and your head rests on your upper arms. Hold and then repeat, re-crossing arms with your opposite arm on top. You can try this same stretch with palms facing down for a slightly different sensation.

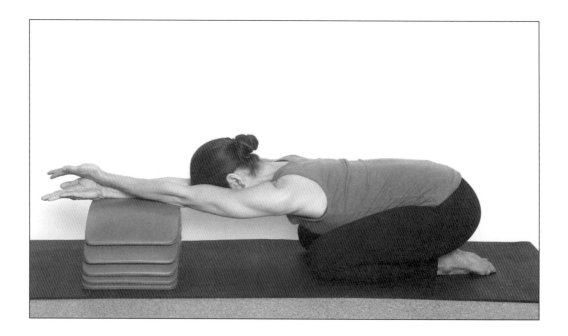

Thread The Needle Stretch

While kneeling, place one arm face down on the Backbridge. Bring your other arm under and across your body, laying it on the mat, palm up. Bring the side of your head or cheek to the mat. Repeat on the opposite side.

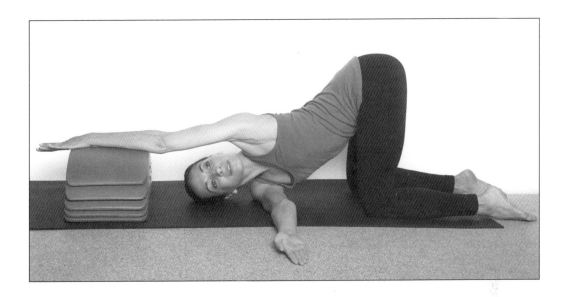

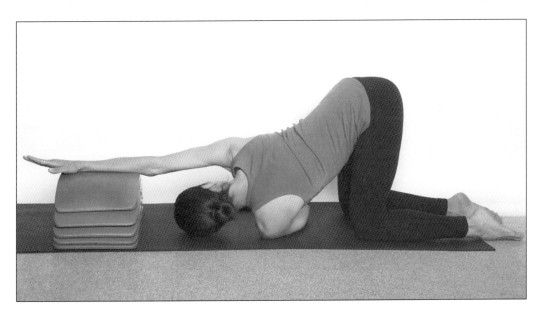

Shoulder And Triceps Stretch

While in the kneeling position, place your elbows on the Backbridge with arms bent at 90 degrees and palms together over your head. Bring buttocks towards your heels.

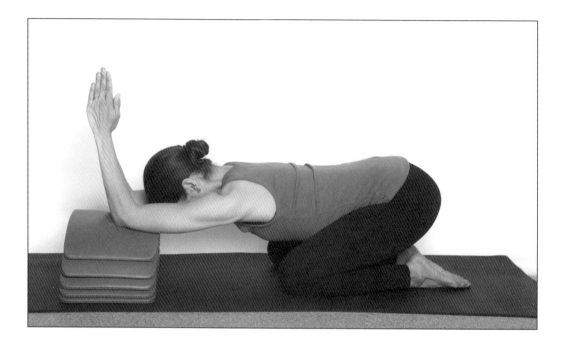

Shoulder Stretches (Face Down)

Lying face down on the mat, place one arm and shoulder on the Backbridge and your other arm in front of you, flat on the floor next to it. Rotate your palm down and hold. Rotate your thumb up and hold. Rotate your palm up and hold. Rotating the placement of your hand will alter the stretch, so you will feel the pull on the sides and backs of your shoulder. Repeat on opposite side.

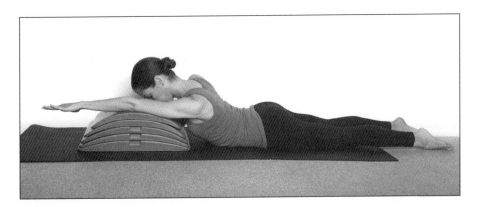

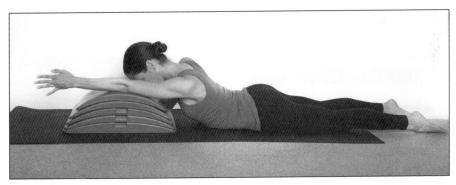

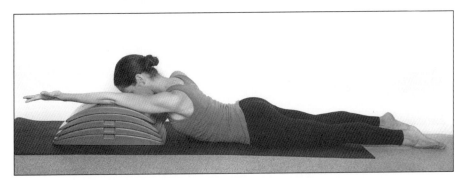

Rotator Cuff Stretch (Pretzel Stretch)

Lie back so that your shoulders are on the highest point of the Backbridge. Bend your arms behind your head, grabbing opposite elbows. Change grip.

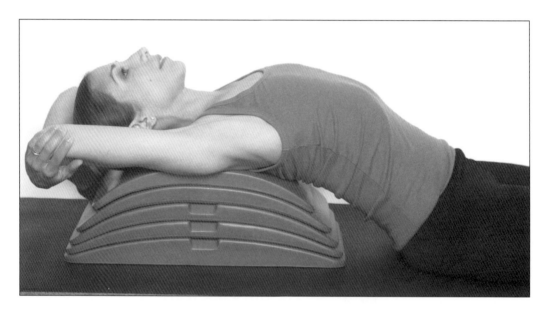

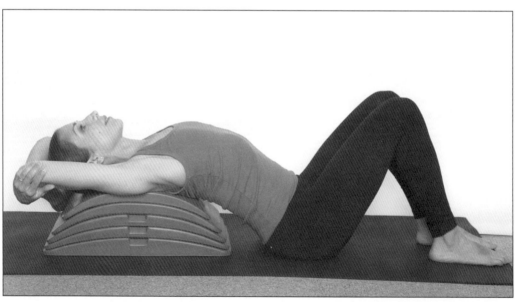

BICEPS AND TRICEPS

The anatomical name for the main biceps muscle is biceps brachii. *Biceps* means "two-headed" and *brachii* means "of the arm," so biceps brachii means "two-headed [muscle] of the arm." The two heads of the biceps connect to different places on the shoulder/scapula region but have a common insertion point on the elbow tendon. This unique structure allows the biceps to carry out their two essential functions:

- ▶ Elbow Flexion, or bending the arm at the elbow joint. An example of this is when you do an arm flex to try to impress your friends.
- ▶ Forearm Supination. Rotating the forearm and hand from side to side. An example of this movement is turning a key to unlock the door.

Another arm muscle typically associated with the biceps muscle group is the lesser-known, but equally important muscle called the brachialis. The brachialis, is located underneath the biceps brachii and assists in the action of elbow flexion.

The anatomical term for your triceps is the triceps brachii. This muscle is located on the back of your upper arm, opposite your biceps. There are three portions of your triceps: the long head, the medial head, and the lateral head. The long head is the part of the muscle that gives you the muscular look when you flex your triceps. The lateral head is next to the long head, closer to the inside of your arm. The medial head is located close to the elbow, at the end of the long and lateral heads. The most important function of the triceps is to straighten the arm.

Biceps Stretch

Sit up straight a few inches in front of the long edge of the Backbridge. Reach back and place your hands on top of the Backbridge with your fingers pointing away from you.

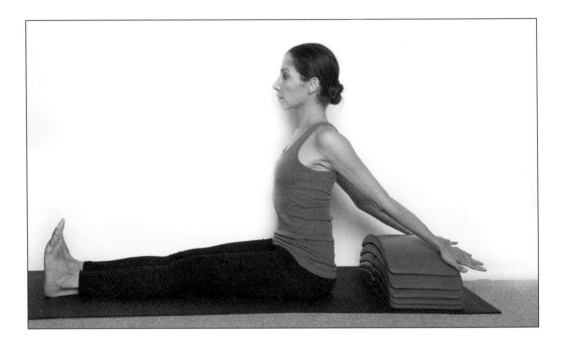

Biceps And Triceps Stretch

From the stretch above, move your hands down so that they are on the ends of the Backbridge. Pull your arms behind you to feel the stretch.

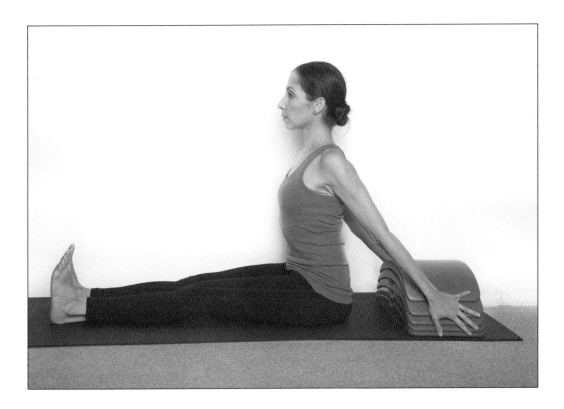

Triceps Stretch

Sit up straight a few inches in front of the long edge of the Backbridge. Reach back and place your hands on top of the Backbridge with your fingers pointing towards you. You can do this with straight or bent arms. You will feel this not only in the triceps but also in the back of your shoulders and your biceps.

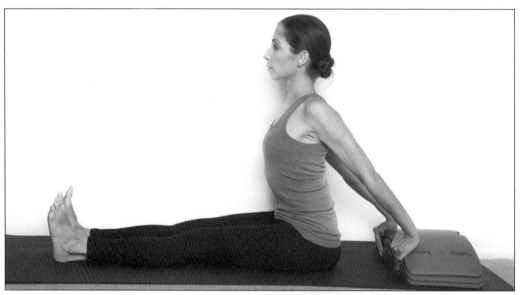

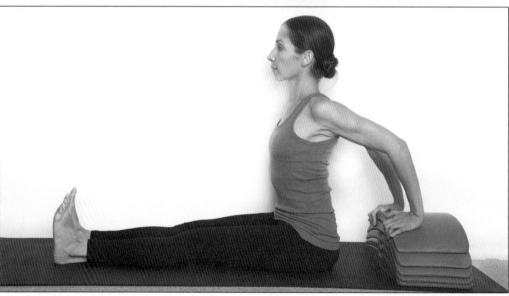

Shoulder And Triceps Stretch

While in the kneeling position, place your elbows on the Backbridge with arms bent at 90 degrees and palms together over your head. Bring your buttocks towards your heels.

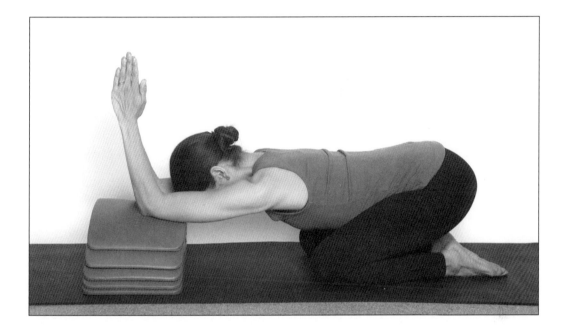

Triceps Stretch (Pretzel Stretch)

Lie back so that your shoulders are on the highest point of the Backbridge. Bend your arms behind your head, grabbing opposite elbows. Change grip.

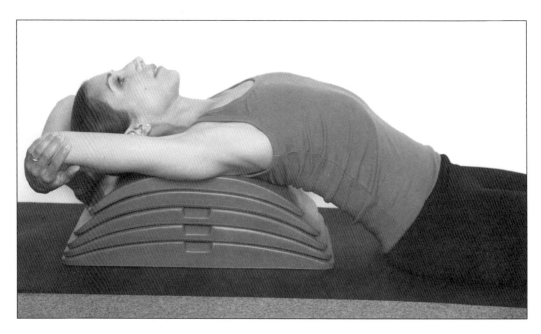

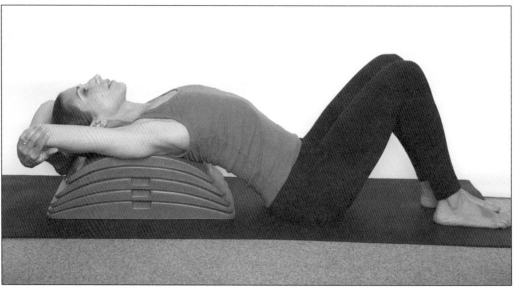

WRIST, FOREARM, AND THUMB

The muscles on the front of the forearm bend your wrist and fingers, and the muscles on the back of the forearm straighten and flex your wrist and fingers. When you are holding things, both groups of muscles work together to stabilize the hands. The following stretches are great for anyone suffering from carpal tunnel, tennis elbow, golfer's elbow or even repetitive strain from computer and phone use. The thumb stretches work on a muscle called the opponens polliciis and help you maintain mobility in your hands.

Wrist And Forearm Stretches

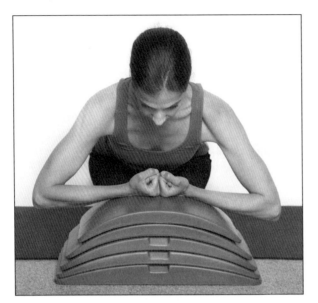

While kneeling on the mat, make two fists and lay the backside of your hands flat on the Backbridge with your fists touching.

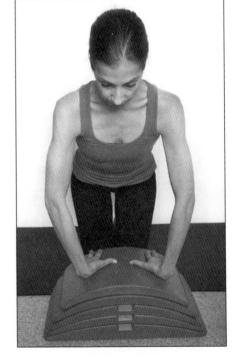

Lie both of your wrists on the Backbridge with your palms up and your fingers facing towards you.

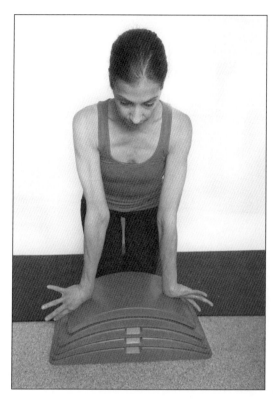

Place the back sides of both your wrists on the Backbridge with your thumbs turned out.

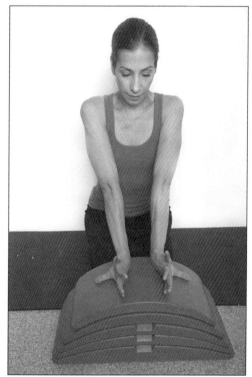

Internally rotate both of your hands and place them on the Backbridge with your thumbs down and pointing away from you.

Place your wrists on the Backbridge, palms facing you, and lean into stretch. If it's more comfortable for you, you can place your the Backbridge on top of a table and lean into the stretch standing up.

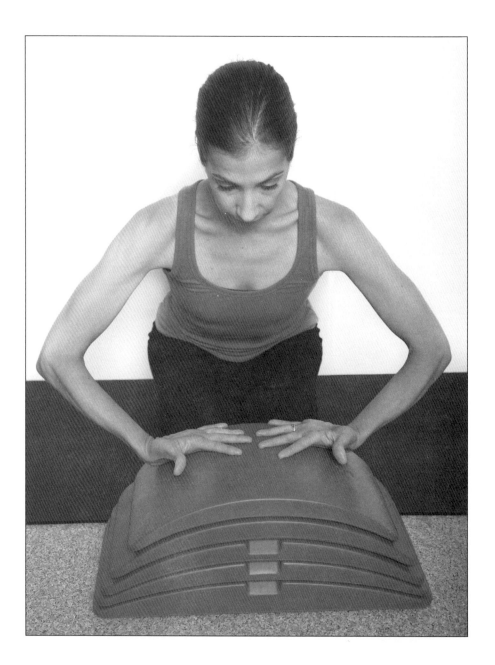

Wrist Stretch

Place the Backbridge with the short end right in front of you. Cross your fingers over one another and place the backs of your wrists on the Backbridge, palms facing you. Lean into your wrists.

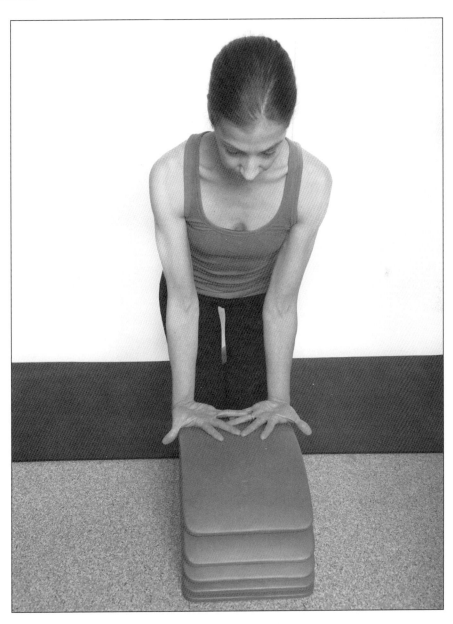

Interior Wrist And Forearm Stretch

Push the Backbridge against a wall to the side of you, about an arm's length away. Then place your hand on the end of the Backbridge. Keeping your arm straight, lean into your wrist. Repeat with other arm.

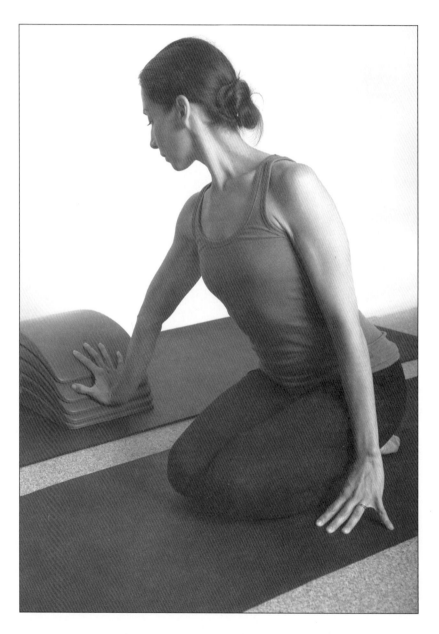

Wrist And Finger Flexor Stretch

Either sitting on your knees or standing with the Backbridge on a tabletop, place both of your hands on the long edges of the Backbridge, turned in towards one another with your palms down. Lean over the Backbridge and slightly bend your elbows, pushing down until you feel the stretch in your wrists and fingers.

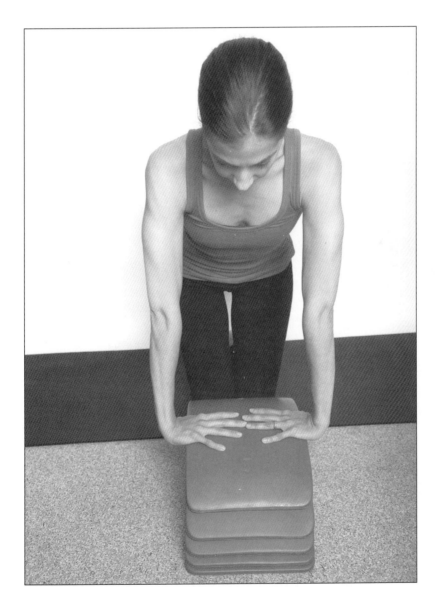

Thumb Stretches

Place both of your thumbs on one long edge of the Backbridge and gently push down.

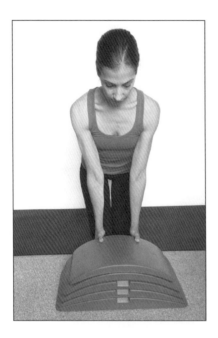

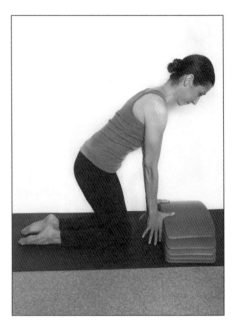

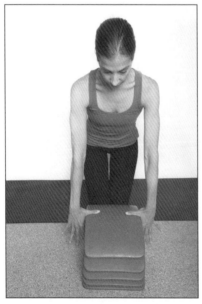

Now place your thumbs on opposite edges of the Backbridge and push into the Backbridge.

NECK AND JAW

Good neck flexibility is important for one's vitality—not to mention the ability to see one's surroundings while driving! Unfortunately, neck pain and discomfort is one of the main reasons patients come to see me. Regardless of the complaint, I check the range of motion in all of my patients' necks because restricted flexibility in the neck can cause a myriad of symptoms, including tight muscles, headaches, dizziness, decreased balance, poor sports performance and even reduced peripheral vision.

Two of the most common misdiagnosed or misunderstood causes of neck tightness are:

1. Too tight abdominal muscles. When we sit, our posture often takes on a forward hunch, causing our abdominals to become shortened and over-contracted, pulling down on the neck and shoulder muscles and creating tremendous pressure. I have included the Backbridge extension stretch as my first neck stretch. While I most certainly understand that this doesn't look like a neck stretch, it releases the abdomen, and its impact on the flexibility of your neck is unparalleled. After two minutes in this stretch, your neck will be much freer in all directions. Check the effectiveness of the stretch simply by seeing how far you can turn your head side to side before and after the stretch.

2. Temporomandibular joint or TMJ dysfunction (jaw tightness). The temporomandibular joint (TMJ) is the area right in front of the ear on either side of the head where the upper jaw (maxilla) and lower jaw (mandible) meet. People frequently clench their teeth, largely as a result of stress. You may not even know you are doing it, whether it be in your sleep or as a coping mechanism during your workday. When the jaw is tight it impacts the neck muscles, resulting in a sore or stiff neck. My simple jaw stretch can help alleviate some of the tension. However, if you continue to have jaw tightness, I recommend trying a night guard that is

sold at the drugstore. Mouth guards can stop some of the harmful effects of clenching and grinding at night. If you find that an over-the-counter mouth guard works for you, you can ask your dentist to custom fit one for long-term use.

The Doctor's Note on Stretching the Neck

Before we begin stretching the neck, it is important to note that the neck moves in several different directions, and I look for good, flexible range of motion in all directions. To check your rotation, which ideally is at 80 degrees, sit up tall and turn your neck to the side. Your chin should line up with your shoulder. Flexion is the act of bringing your chin to your chest, and lateral flexion is your ability to bring your ear to your shoulder. To qualify as having "good flexibility," you should be able to touch your chin to your chest and move your head about 25 degrees, or halfway, to the shoulder. Extension is the ability to bring your head back, optimally about 55 degrees. You should always check extension while sitting, as some may get dizzy while standing. The neck can move in a combination of these directions at the same time, such as laterally bending and rotating. When stretching the neck, you want to be very careful not to overstretch, which can cause painful neck spasms.

In order to best protect the neck, I like to do passive neck stretches and then restricted stretches with the stretch strap. The passive stretches just move your neck through its range of motion; the restrictive stretches allow us to move our neck up against slight resistance created by the strap. Do the passive stretches first to make sure that you are ready to add some resistance from the stretch strap. Remember, stretching should never hurt!

The Backbridge Extension

Sit at the base of the Backbridge. Lie back so that the highest point of the Backbridge is between your shoulder blades and your head touches the floor. Rest your arms behind your head and hold this stretch for 2 minutes. Level 1 is the easiest and 5 is the hardest. Pick a level that is most comfortable for you. It should feel like a good stretch. After a few weeks, slowly progress to the next level.

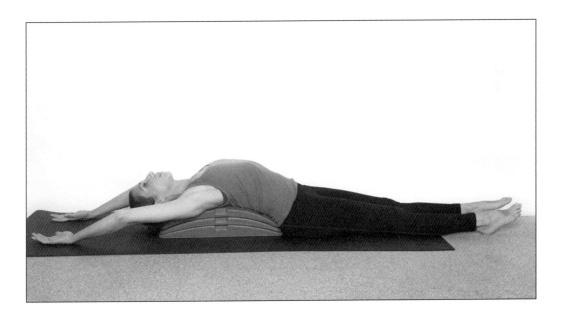

Side Neck Stretch

Sit in a comfortable cross-legged position on the Backbridge. Take your right hand and place it above your left ear, fingers pointing down. Your left hand can rest on your left thigh. Begin to gently pull your head, bringing your right ear towards the top of your right shoulder until you feel a stretch in the left side of your neck. Repeat on the other side.

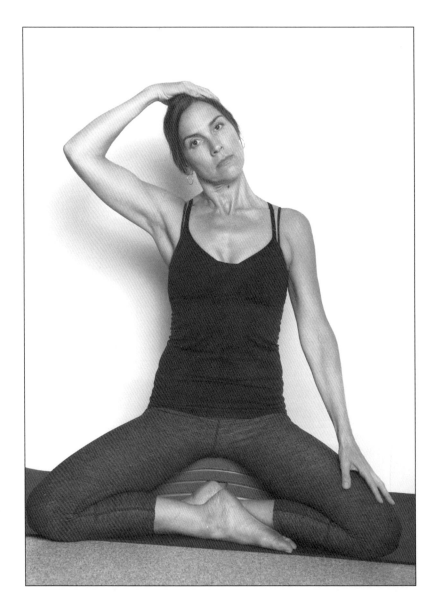

Side Neck Stretch With Upward Tilt

While sitting comfortably on the Backbridge, take your left hand and place it palm down on the top, right side of your head. Gently pull your head on a diagonal back and to the left, bringing your chin up and to the right. You should feel this stretch on the right, front side of your neck. Repeat on the other side.

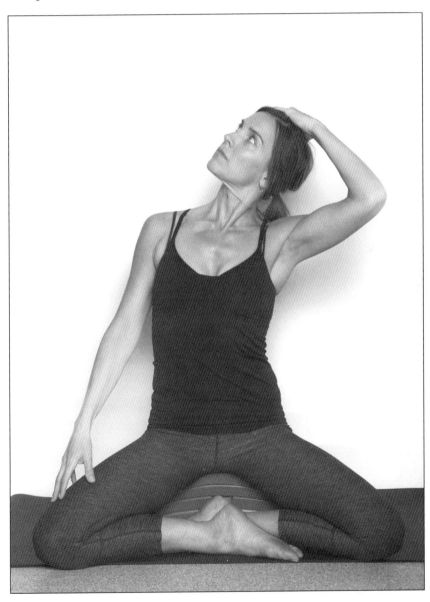

Side Neck Rotation Stretch

While seated on the Backbridge, take your left fingertips and place them on the right side of your chin. Keeping your head neutral (with your chin parallel to the floor), begin to gently turn your head to the left with your chin facing your left shoulder. You should feel a comfortable stretch in the right side of your neck. Repeat on the other side.

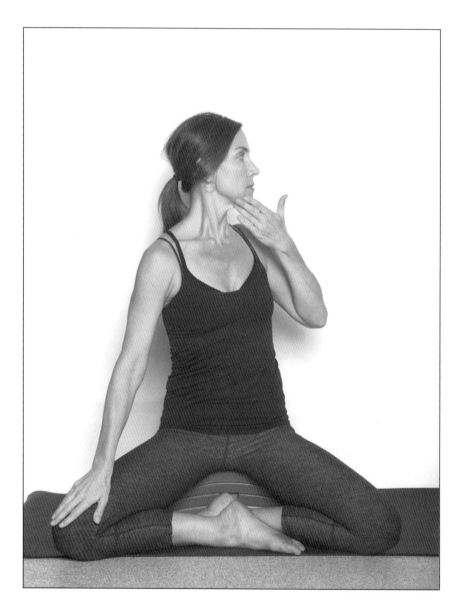

Side/Back Of Neck Stretch

Remain in your comfortable seat on the Backbridge. Take your left hand and place it on top of your head with your fingers pointing down toward the back, right side of your neck. Begin to gently pull your head forward and down on a diagonal as if you were bringing your chin towards your right shoulder. Repeat on the other side.

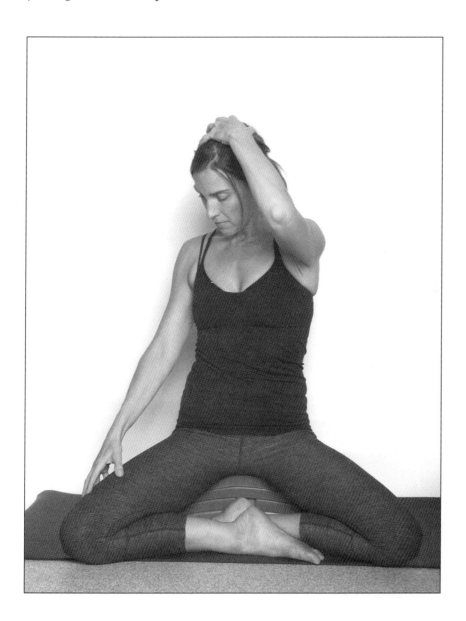

Front Of Neck Stretch

Bend your elbows to the side and place both of your hands behind your head with fingertips touching or interlaced. If your shoulders are very tight and you cannot relax them in this position, you may also use a strap to support your neck as shown below. Gently tilt your head straight back until you feel a comfortable stretch in the front of your neck.

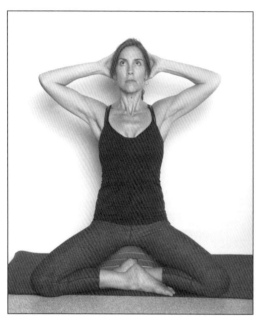 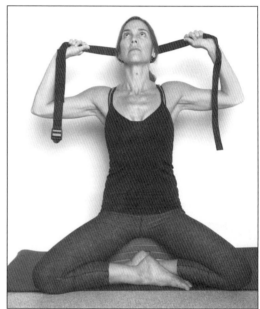

Back of Neck Stretch

Keep the same hand (or strap) position as the previous stretch. You may also try placing the strap across your forehead if this position is more comfortable for your shoulders and/or neck. Drop your chin and allow your head to bow forward, creating a comfortable stretch in the back of the neck.

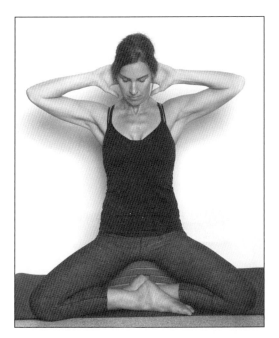
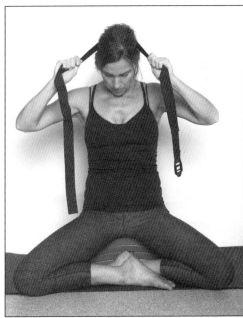

Jaw Stretch

Place your fingertips just inside the jaw joint (next to your ears) and apply gentle pressure while you slowly open and close your mouth, raising and lowering the jaw bone or mandible. Do this 10 times, pause, and repeat.

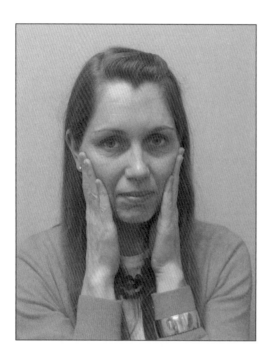 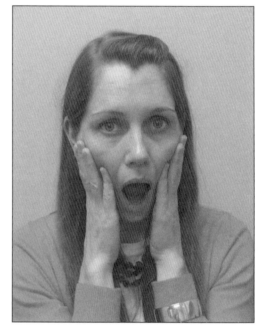

4

Tandem Stretching

T andem or partner stretching is rooted in resistance flexibility and is a great way to increase the intensity of a stretch. It also helps the person performing the stretch maintain good form. This section contains partner stretches that can be done on the floor or lying on a table. Just remember to communicate with your partner to avoid over-stretching or injuries!

Leg Distraction

Lay over the Backbridge with your buttocks on the highest point and have your stretch partner gently pull your outstretched legs towards him/her. This is a great stretch to relieve pressure on the lower back and spinal discs. Make sure that the person being stretched remains on the Backbridge and doesn't slide. The higher the level of the Backbridge you use, the greater the stretch you will feel.

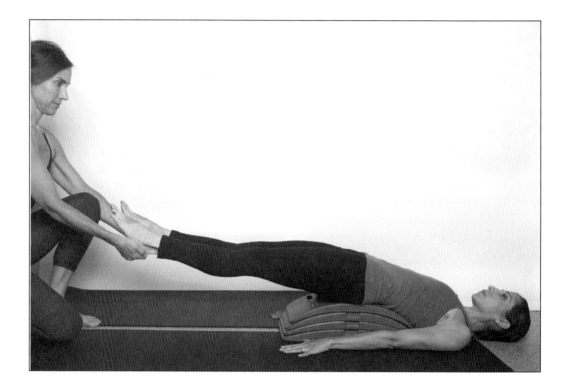

Arm Distraction

Using the same positioning as the leg distraction, raise your arms above your head. Your stretch partner will gently pull your wrists away from you and towards them. This stretch will also decompress and elongate the spine. If this stretch bothers your wrists, have your partner hold your forearms.

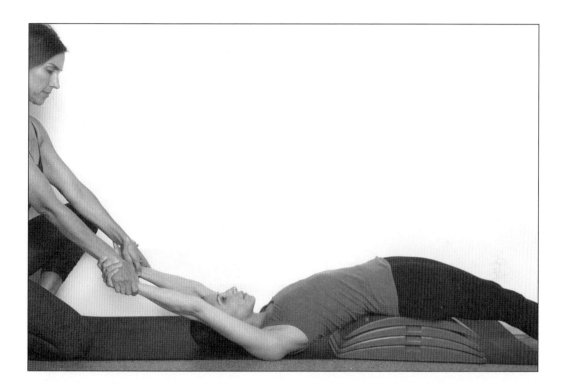

Hamstring And Hip Flexor Stretch

From the last stretches, raise one leg straight up in the air while the opposite leg is extended out straight on the mat. Your stretch partner will gently push your raised leg toward you while gently applying downward pressure on the thigh of the opposite, outstretched leg. The higher the level of the Backbridge you use, the greater the range of motion and the deeper the stretch. Switch legs and repeat.

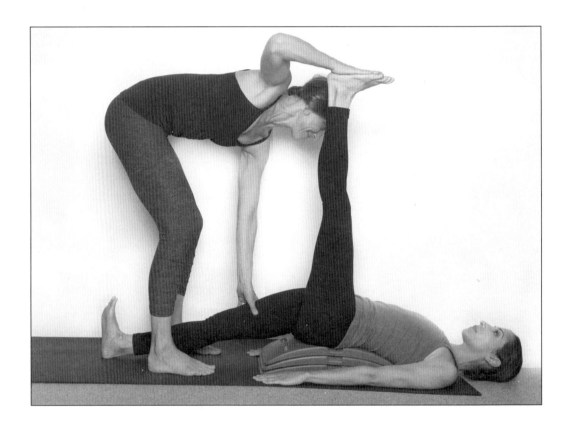

Knees To Chest Stretch

Lay over the Backbridge with your buttocks on the hightest point. Bring your knees to your chest. Your stretch partner will place downward pressure on your shins to increase the stretch on your hip flexors and lower back.

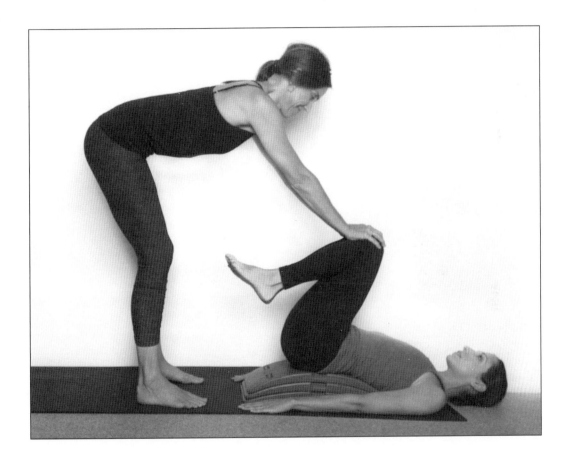

Single Knee To Chest Stretch

From the last stretch, bend one knee to your chest while you extend the opposite leg straight out on the mat. Your partner will gently apply pressure just below your bent knee, bringing it closer to your chest while also applying downward pressure on the opposite, outstretched leg. Switch legs and repeat.

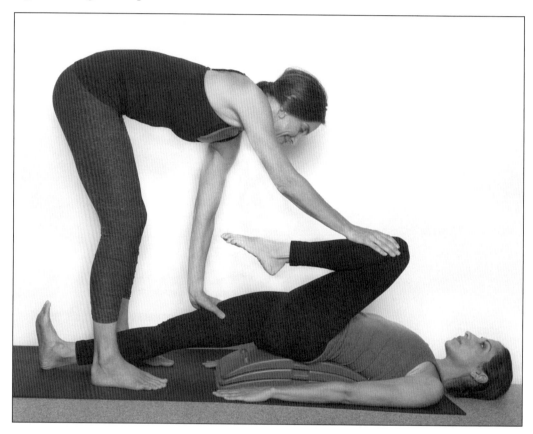

Piriformis Stretch

From the last stretch, cross one knee over the other in a figure 4 position (you can do this with two bent legs or one straight leg.) Your stretch partner will gradually move your legs closer to your chest to increase the stretch in your piriformis. Switch legs and repeat.

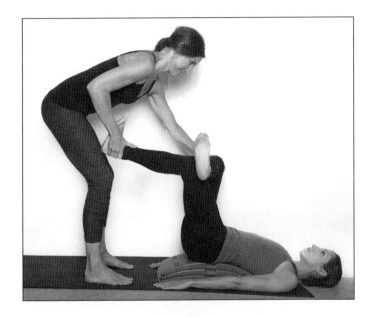

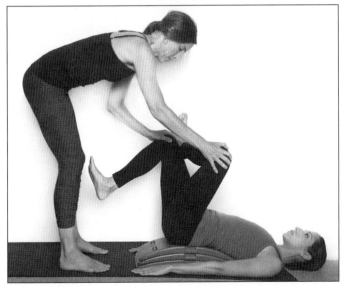

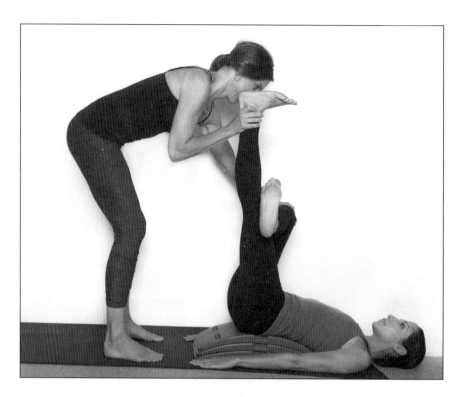

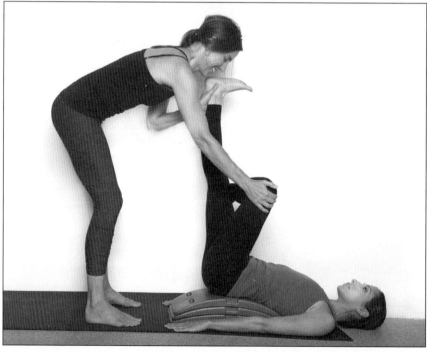

Groin And Lumbar Stretch

Place the Backbridge on the floor, and sit on the highest point with legs spread in a "V." Keeping your back as straight as possible, hinge at hips and extend your arms in front of you. Your stretch partner will gently pull your wrists towards them. You will feel a nice stretch through your groin and lower back.

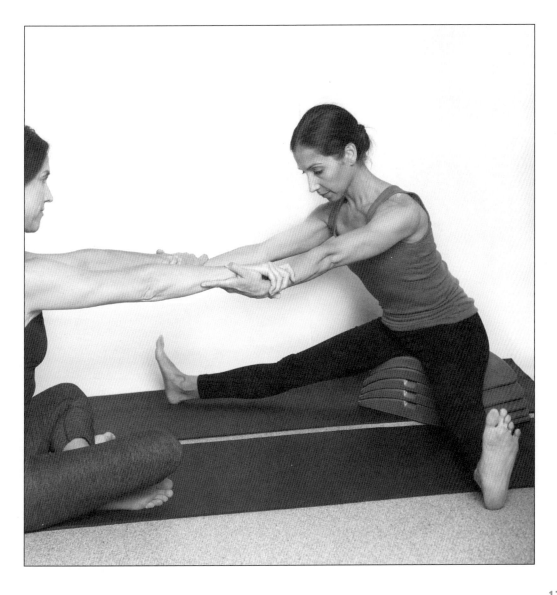

Lumbar Paraspinal Stretch

From the previous stretch, place your hands or forearms in front of you on the mat with your elbows bent. Your partner will gently push forward and down on your low back to increase the stretch.

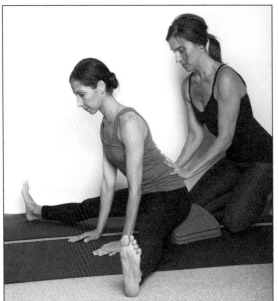

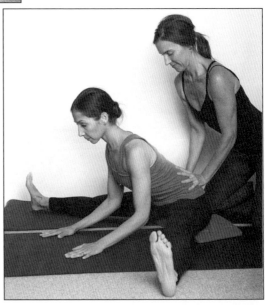

5

Balance or Proprioception

The term proprioception, more commonly known as balance, refers to the ability to sense and continually adapt to where you are in space. A high level of balance allows you to respond to your environment more quickly and effectively, decreasing your risk of injury. For example, the football receiver who is able to jump in the air, contort his body to make a catch, and make a stable landing shows high proprioception, or excellent balance.

Balance exercises will allow you to engage your core, stabilize your muscles and align your body. Balance and coordination are vital pieces in obtaining optimum health and fitness, but are unfortunately frequently ignored. Practicing these balance poses can dramatically improve your quality of life by allowing you to become more limber and less susceptible to injury. These specific functional exercises will also challenge your nervous system and ultimately improve your performance in sports or other fitness activities.

A frequent cause of repeated ankle sprains, for example, is not necessarily from weakened ankle muscles, but from the loss of proprioceptive or balance responders. How is this so? Well, the body has a sensory motor system, which acts like a master computer. The ankle, for instance, sends feedback to your brain, telling the brain where it is. The brain, in turn, responds, telling the ankle what to do. When injury happens to the ankle, a little bit of the communication between the brain and the ankle is lost, not only causing inflammation and irritation to the ankle, but also reducing its proprioceptive response. For areas of the body that have a large balance response, like the foot or the ankle, it is imperative that we improve or rehabilitate that proprioceptive response to prevent future delay in the communication and, therefore, injury. Those who think they have weak ankles or a bad knee may, in fact, just have a poor proprioceptive response. Doing these balance exercise will improve your proprioceptive response, thus reducing the frequency of ankle sprains or similar injuries.

Simply put, these balance stretches will heighten your awareness of where everything is at all times and help you be more in control of your body. You will be able to bend over, balance on one leg and move your body in many different positions with greater ease and less chance of injury.

Again, the great thing about the Backbridge is its ability to make these balance exercises easier or harder by adding or subtracting different levels. For most of these balance exercises, the more levels under your feet, the greater the instability, making the exercise harder. Remember, the Backbridge is all about progression and having the ability to alter the intensity of the balance stretches and poses while continually challenging your body and nervous system.

Side Leg Balance

Stand with your left foot in the center of level 1 of the Backbridge (the Backbridge can be either parallel or perpendicular to your body). You can either keep your right foot hovering just above the mat, or raise it out to the side to increase the balance challenge. Place your hands on your hips or raise your arms out to the side to assist your balance. Switch legs and repeat.

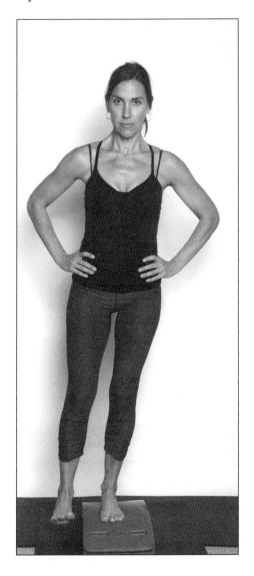 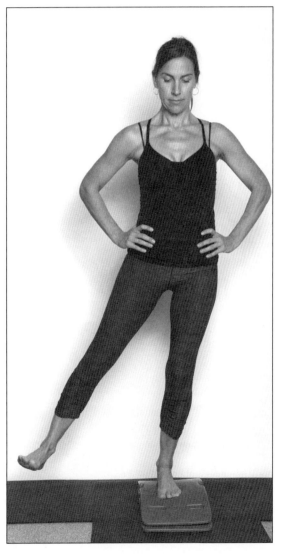

Side Leg Raises

Using the same position as the previous exercise, lift your non-standing leg out to the side and then lower it to hover just above the mat or the Backbridge. Repeat 10 times and switch legs.

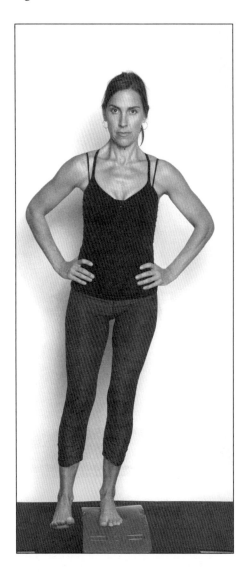 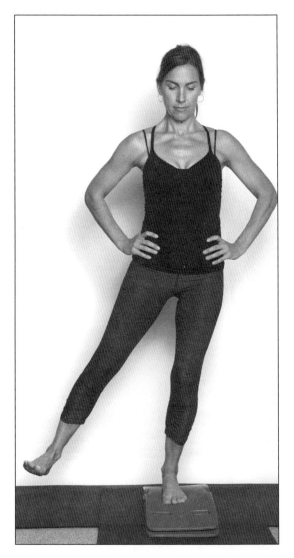

Front Leg Balance And Raises (Straight Leg)

Remain in the same position, now raising one leg straight out in front of you. You can either hold this position and balance or do a set of 10 leg raises, trying to keep the foot that is raised from touching down during the repetitions. Switch legs and repeat.

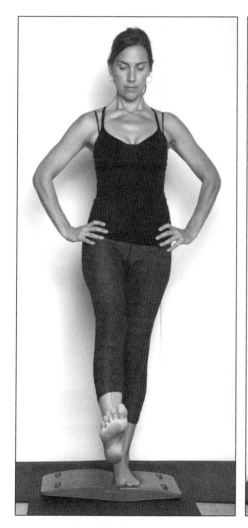
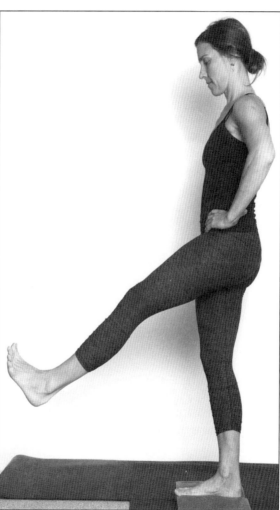

Front Leg Balance And Raise (With Bent Knee)

Standing on one foot in the center of the Backbridge, raise your other leg in front of you, bending at the knee so your leg is at a 90 degree angle. You can stay here and balance, or do 10 repetitions of raising and lowering your knee, keeping your foot off the mat the entire time. Switch legs and repeat.

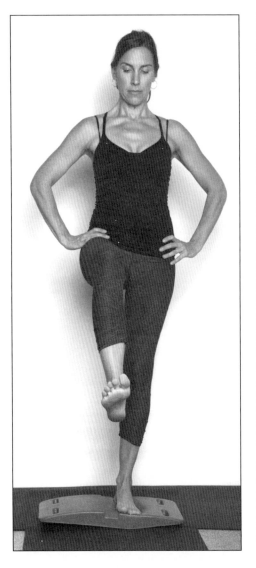
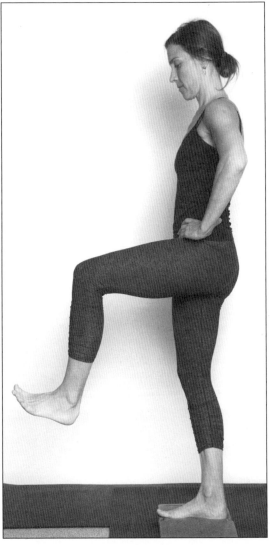

Tree Pose Balance

This traditional yoga pose can be practiced using the Backbridge to introduce an instability factor. Stand with your left foot in the center of the Backbridge, level 1. Bending your right knee and externally rotating your right leg from the hip, place the ball of your right foot on the Backbridge. Your toes and right knee will point out to the right. For increased difficulty (and an increased hip opening stretch), bring the sole of your right foot to the inside of your left calf, just below your left knee or to the inside of your thigh, just above the knee. Never place your foot directly on the side of your knee as this can create harmful pressure on the joint. Place your hands on your hips for balance or raise your arms above your head for an increased challenge. Switch legs and repeat.

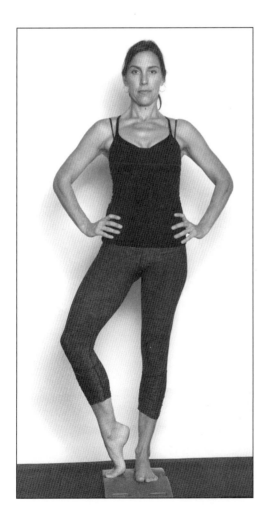 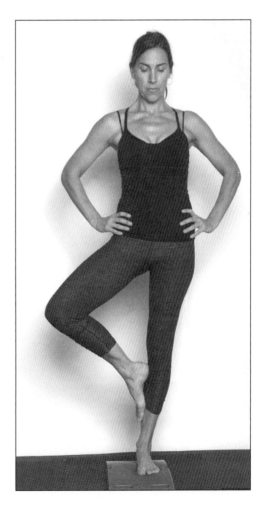

Warrior 3 Balance Pose

Standing with your left foot on the center of the Backbridge, slowly lean forward while simultaneously raising your right leg behind you. Keep your hips square and pointing forward as you reach out through your right leg, keeping your right foot flexed with the toes pointing down. As your balance improves in this exercise, work toward keeping both legs straight and leaning further forward in this pose. You can keep the arms straight and close to your sides with palms facing forward/down or you can bring the arms out to a "T" to assist with the balance. Switch legs and repeat.

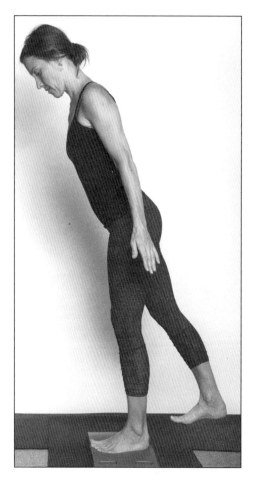
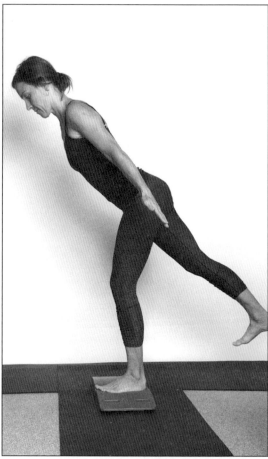

6

Yoga with the Backbridge

Yoga is a great way to stretch and relax your mind, body and muscles. You may be familiar with a traditional yoga block, which makes poses (or asanas) easier or more accessible for those who are either new to yoga or have a limited range of motion caused by tight muscles or natural anatomical structure. Yoga blocks can also serve as an extension of your arms to facilitate and/or improve alignment in certain poses. the Backbridge is a replacement for a yoga block and is actually a better prop in many asanas because it is more comfortable, more stable and better contoured to fit your body.

Yoga blocks come at only one standard height, while the five different levels of your Backbridge allow for many alterations, so that you can make different poses either easier or harder, depending on your flexibility and yoga experience. For a beginner in yoga, the Backbridge can make the practice safer and easier by supporting your body and reducing the potential for one to overstretch. For the expert, the Backbridge can maximize certain muscle groups' isolation, allowing for a deeper stretch. Adding and taking away the Backbridge levels allows the user to progress at his/her own rate and modify on days of tightness or soreness. the Backbridge can also help all yogis maintain proper form and alignment throughout their practice.

Remember, yoga is not about pain or competition. It's about being aware of your own body, and stretching it mindfully. With its stackable levels, the Backbridge allows for a more tailored yoga practice and offers more options to grow in the poses.

Balasana (Child's Pose)

Kneel on the floor in front of the Backbridge. Touch your big toes together and separate your knees about as wide as your hips. Sitting back on your heels, bring your torso toward your knees and rest your forehead on the Backbridge. You can either lay your hands on the floor alongside your torso, palms up, or reach out and extend your arms forward with your palms face down on the mat. Level 1 of the Backbridge allows for the deepest stretch, but those with knee pain or injury may find that such a deep knee flex bothers the joints. For these practitioners, level 5 will be most comfortable.

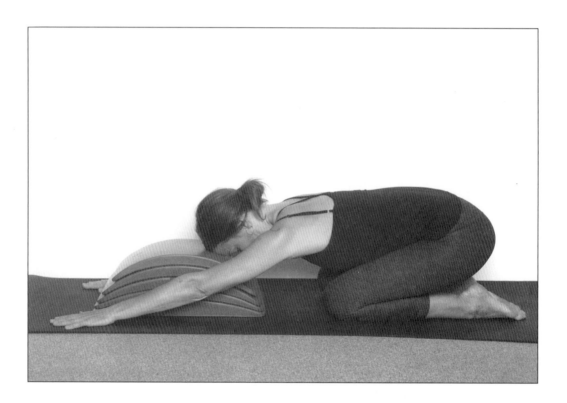

Marjaryasana (Cat Pose) and Bitilasana (Cow Pose)

With the Backbridge perpendicular to your body, kneel on level 1 or 2 of the Backbridge, which allows for extra cushion underneath the knees and creates a more comfortable practice. Bring your hands to the floor in "tabletop" position, making sure your knees are set directly below your hips and your wrists are directly under your shoulders. Center your head in a neutral position, eyes looking at the floor. As you exhale, round your spine toward the ceiling, making sure to keep your shoulders and knees in position. Release your head toward the floor, but don't force your chin to your chest. As you inhale, lift your sitting bones and chest toward the ceiling, allowing your belly to sink toward the floor. Repeat this movement of cat and cow about 10 times, following the rhythm of your breath.

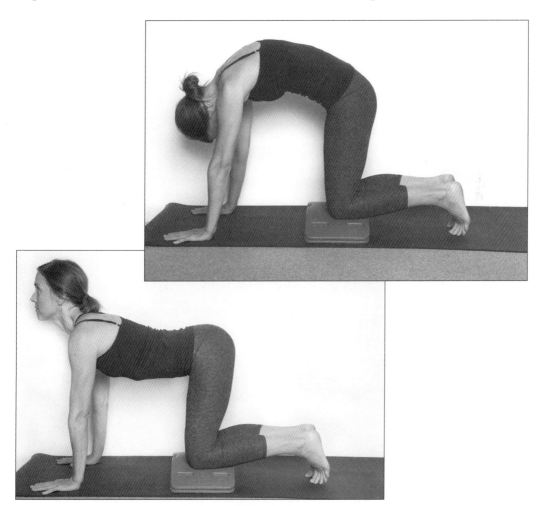

Anjaneyasana (Crescent Lunge)

From Cat/Cow, turn the Backbridge so that it is now parallel with your body. Kneel on the highest point of the Backbridge and step your right foot forward, bending your leg at 90 degrees (your knee should be directly over your ankle). Place your hands on top of your right knee or raise your arms overhead with your biceps next to your ears. Hold this pose for several rounds of breath and repeat on the other side. Level 1 is suggested for the deepest stretch, offering cushion for the knee cap as well as increased stability, which ensures more effective posture. Adding levels decreases the depth of the lunge and the amount of opening in the hip flexor, making the stretch easier for those who need modification.

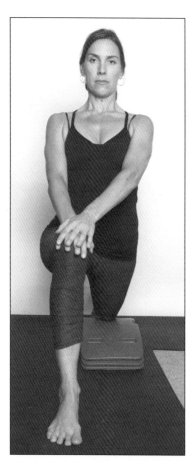

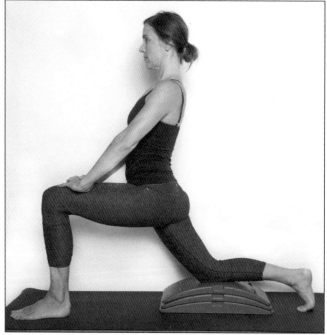

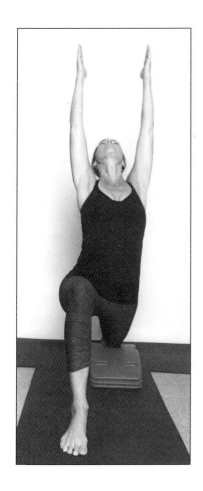

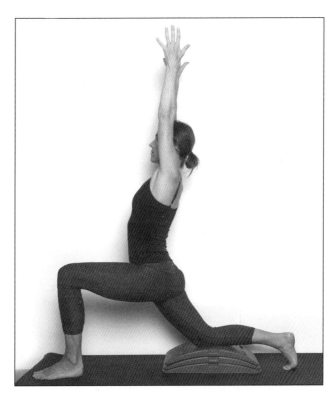

Virabhadrasana III (Warrior III Pose)

Coming out of crescent lunge, place the Backbridge perpendicular to you about six to twelve inches in front of your right foot and put your hands on top. Slowly begin to straighten the right leg while you simultaneously lift the left leg straight behind you until it is parallel to the floor. Keep the left foot flexed with the toes pointing down and both hips square with the ground. Keep the back of your neck long with your gaze at your hands or just in front of the Backbridge. Stay here for about 30 seconds, keeping both legs active and engaged. Slowly begin to bend the right leg, returning the left foot to the mat. Switch legs and repeat.

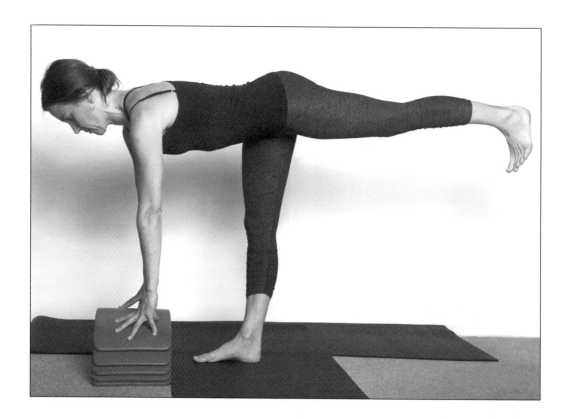

Parivrtta Utkatasana (Revolved Chair Pose)

Stand just behind the long edge of the Backbridge with your feet together. Raise your arms straight out to the sides. Slowly bend your knees so that they are directly over your toes and fold forward at the waist, as if you were sitting in a chair. Twisting at your waist, rotate your torso to the left, bringing your right hand to the top of the Backbridge and extending your left arm up to the ceiling. Your right knee may tend to pop forward here, so be sure to draw your right hip back to keep it in line with the left knee. Stay here for 15 to 30 seconds and then unwind. Twist to the opposite side.

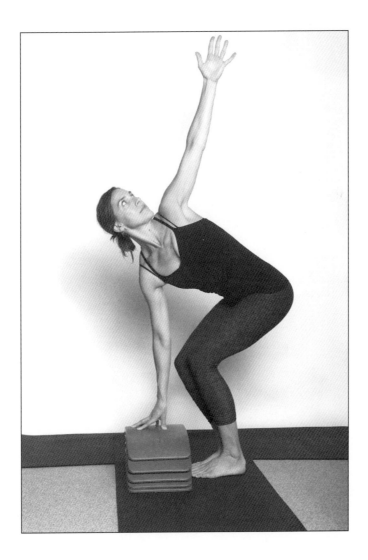

Bhujangasana (Cobra Pose)

Lying face down over the Backbridge with your belly button near the highest point, place your hands in front of you and do half a push up so that your upper torso is elevated but your pelvis still has contact with the Backbridge. Look straight ahead or raise your eyes to the ceiling and hold for several breaths, then slowly lower yourself down and repeat. This stretch really works your lumbar extenders and lower back while stretching and lengthening the core (abdominals). The higher the level of the Backbridge you use, the easier the stretch will be.

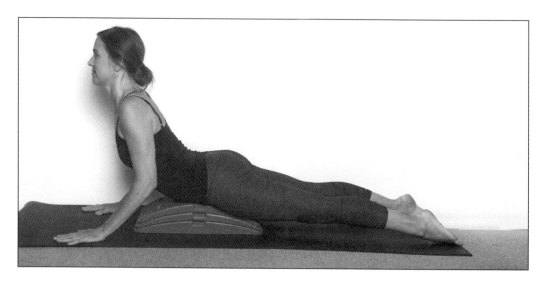

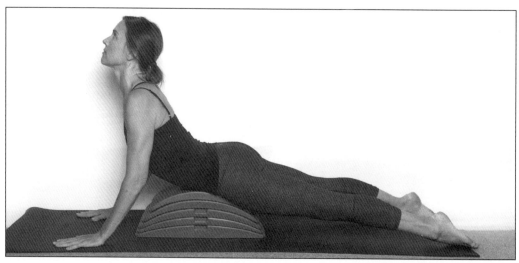

Salabhasana (Locust Pose)

Lay over the Backbridge again, but now straighten your arms and clasp your hands behind your back. On an inhale, gently lift your head and chest off the mat, reaching back toward your heels with your clasped hands. Hold for several breaths and slowly lower your upper body to the mat. Repeat 2-3 times. You'll feel this stretch in your back and arms.

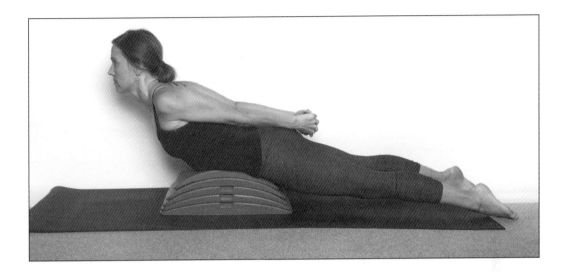

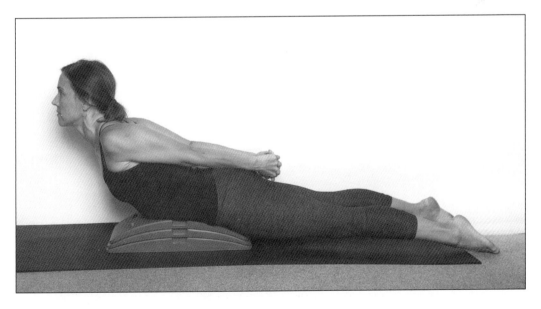

Dhanurasana (Bow Pose)

For a more intense backbend, lie on your belly over the Backbridge with your hands alongside your torso, palms up. Bend your knees and bring your heels toward your buttocks. Reach back and hold the outsides of your ankles with the thumbs facing down toward the mat. You can try this pose with flexed or pointed feet. On an inhale, reach your heels away from your buttocks, lifting your torso up off the mat. Extend your tailbone toward the floor while you contract your shoulder blades to open your chest. Draw the tops of the shoulders away from your ears and look forward. Stay in this pose for several breaths, feeling the stretch in your back, your chest, and the front of your thighs, and then gently lower down, releasing your feet. Using level 5 is the easiest, giving you more support and decreasing your range of motion. As your range of motion increases you can remove levels, giving you a deeper stretch.

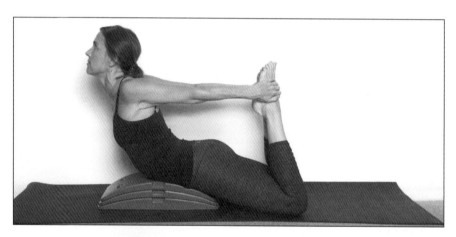

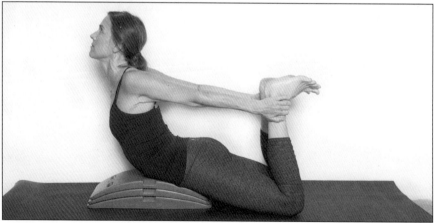

Ustrasana (Camel Pose)

Kneel on the Backbridge, knees hip width apart and thighs perpendicular to the floor. Place your hands on your low back with your fingers pointing up or down and your elbows bent. Lean back slightly, keeping your thighs perpendicular to the floor. For more advanced practitioners, reach your hands back to grab your heels. Hold this pose for several breaths, feeling the stretch in your back as you relieve the day's forward flexion. Use level 1 or 2 of the Backbridge for knee cushion and comfort. Going higher may compromise the safety and alignment of the backbend.

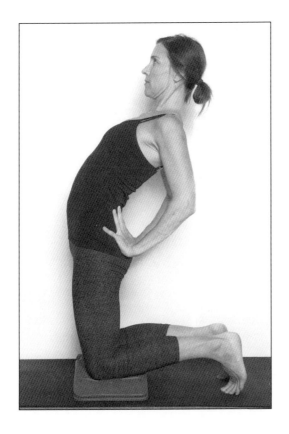
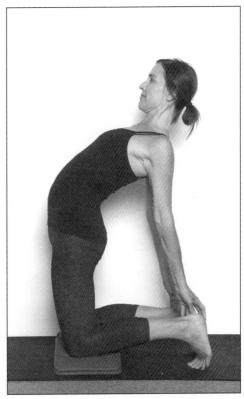

Virasana (Hero Pose)

Start in kneeling position and sit back on top of the Backbridge, with the front of both shins and the top of both feet on the mat underneath you. the Backbridge makes this pose easier, so enjoy the resting pose before moving into the following variation.

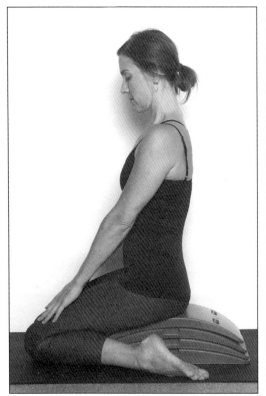
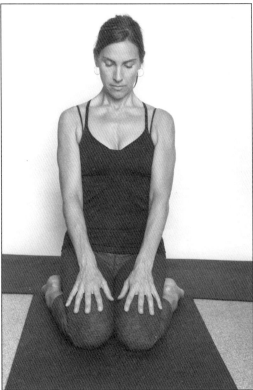

Gomukhasana (Cow Face Pose) In Hero Pose

Sitting on the Backbridge in hero pose, inhale and stretch your right arm straight out to the side, parallel to the floor. Rotate your arm so your thumb turns toward the floor. As you exhale, bring your upper arm in, so that it is flush against your side. Put your forearm behind you on your low back. Roll your shoulder back and down, gently working your forearm up your back until it is parallel to your spine. The back of your hand will ideally be between your shoulder blades. Reach your left arm up and over your head. Bending your elbow, lower your arm behind your head and rotate your palm to face your back with your thumb pointing to the left. Bring your left hand to touch the right hand, hooking the right and left fingers if possible. If you can't reach, use a strap. Hold the pose for several breaths and repeat on other side.

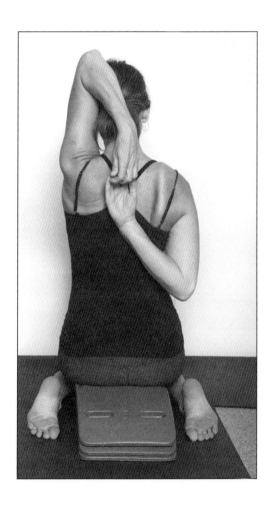 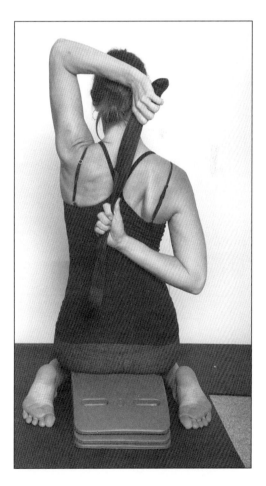

Eka Pada Rajakapotasana (Pigeon Pose)

Place your Backbridge next to you on the mat on level 1, 2 or 3. Begin on hands and knees in a tabletop position, with your knees directly below your hips, and your hands below your shoulders. Bring your right knee forward to the back of your right wrist, and your right foot toward your left wrist so that your shin is parallel to, and resting on, the mat. Keeping your right foot flexed, slowly slide your left leg back, straightening the knee and bringing the top of the thigh to the floor. Square your hips to the front of the mat. Pull the Backbridge in under your right buttock and lower yourself to the top of the Backbridge. Stay in this position and breathe, feeling the opening in the outside of your right hip. Bend your left knee, bringing your left heel toward your left buttock. Reach your left arm back and grab the inside or outside of the left ankle or foot, keeping your chest lifted. Alternately, you can raise your left arm up and bending the elbow, grab the left foot (option to use both hands on the strap). Hold for several breaths, feeling the stretch along the outer right hip and the top of the left thigh. Gently release your left foot back to the mat. Repeat on the other side.

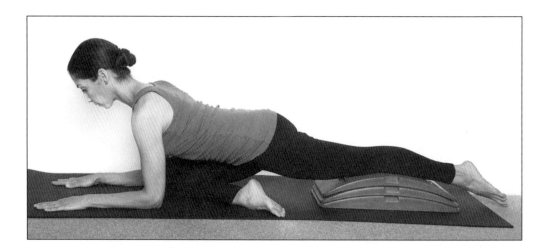

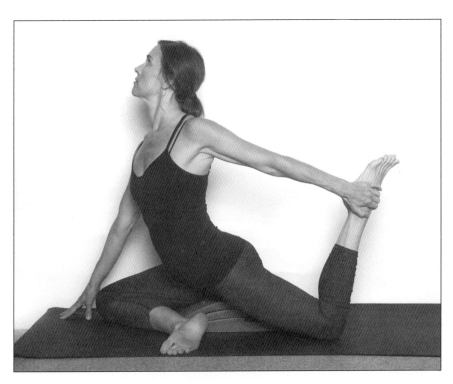

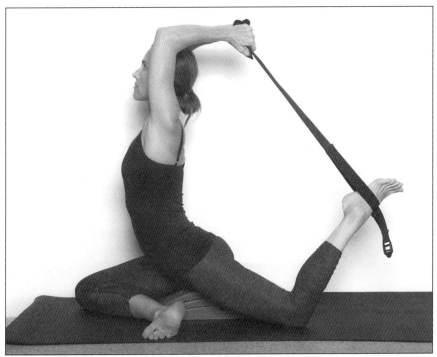

Ardha Matsyendrasana (Half Lord Of The Fishes Pose)

Sit on the Backbridge with your legs straight out in front of you. Bend your knees and bring your left foot under your right leg to the outside of your right hip, laying the left leg on the mat. If this is too much for your hips, you can extend your left leg out straight along the mat in front of you. Step your right foot over the left thigh, placing it just outside of your left thigh so that the knee is pointing to the ceiling. With a straight arm, place your right hand on the Backbridge just behind your right buttock. Bending your left arm, twist your torso to the right and place the outside of your left elbow on the outside of your right knee. Inhale and lengthen your torso. Exhale and deepen the twist. Repeat for several breaths and then switch legs and twist to the opposite side.

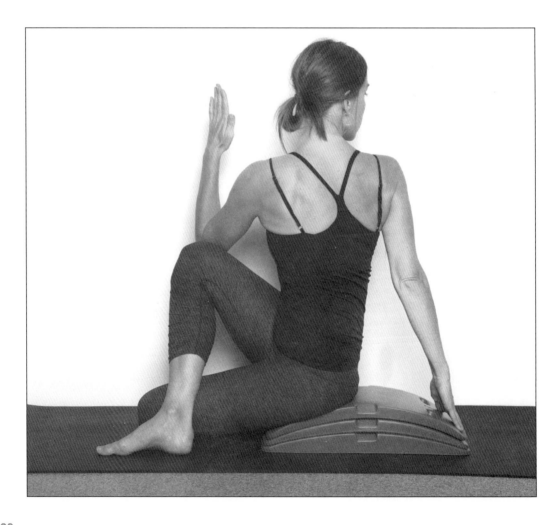

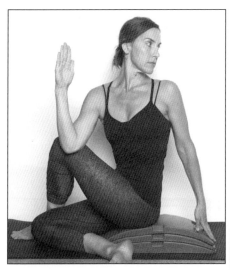

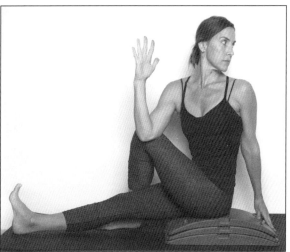

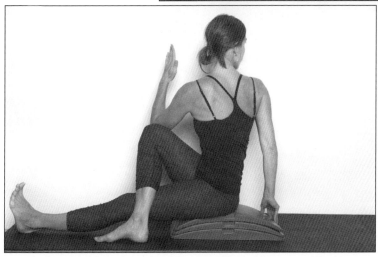

Utthita Trikonasana (Extended Triangle Pose)

Step your right leg forward on the mat, so that it is about three to four feet in front of, and slightly to the right of, the left foot with toes pointing forward. Rotate the left foot almost 90 degrees so it is close to perpendicular to the back edge of your mat. The heel of your right foot should be aligned with arch of your left foot. Place the Backbridge on the mat just to the outside of your right shin. Extend your arms to each side so they are parallel with the ground, and hinge forward from the front hip over the right thigh. Place your right hand on top of the Backbridge and revolve the bottom ribs up towards the ceiling, your gaze straight ahead or up toward the top (left) hand. Stay in the pose for several breaths. From here you can move to Ardha Chandrasana and Parivrtta Ardha Chandrasana (both following) or on an inhale, maintain length through the torso and keep the legs engaged, coming up the same way you came into the pose.

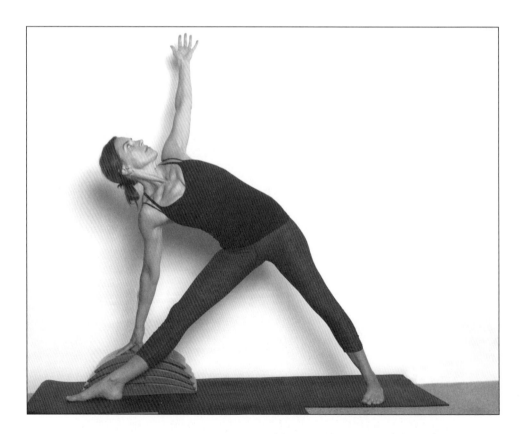

Ardha Chandrasana (Half Moon Pose)

From triangle pose on the right side, bring your left hand to rest on the left hip. Move the Backbridge in front of your right foot, and bending your right knee, slide your left foot about 6 to 12 inches forward along the floor. Reach your right hand forward and place it on the Backbridge. Press your right foot firmly into the floor, and straighten your right leg while lifting the left leg until it is parallel to the floor. Stay active in both legs, keeping the raised foot flexed. Advanced practitioners may extend the left arm up to the ceiling. Stay in the pose for several breaths, then move to Parivrtta Ardha Chandrasana (following) or lower the raised left leg to the mat and return to Trikonasana.

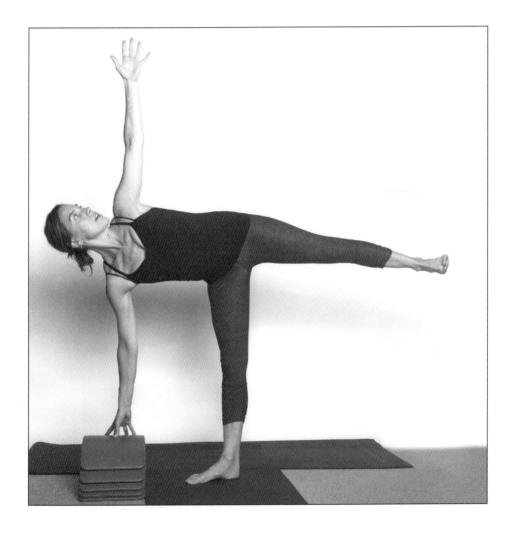

Parivrtta Ardha Chandrasana (Revolved Half Moon Pose)

From Half Moon Pose, revolve your torso and hips so that they point towards the floor, bringing your right hand to the top of the Backbridge. Keeping your right leg raised with your foot flexed and your toes pointing down, slowly begin to twist your torso to the left, bringing your left hand to your left hip or raising your arm to the ceiling. Stay here and breathe for 30 seconds. To come out of the pose, bring your left hand back to the Backbridge and slowly lower your right leg to the mat. Repeat sequence of three poses on the other side.

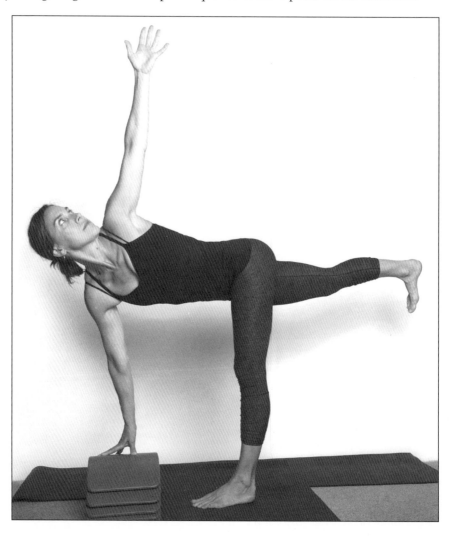

Parivrtta Trikonasana (Revolved Triangle Pose)

Begin standing with your feet in the same position as triangle pose, with the right foot forward and the left foot about a leg's length behind. Place the Backbridge outside of your right foot. Turn your torso to the right, so that your hips face forward. Raise your arms out to the side, parallel to the ground, then, turn your torso further to the right and lean forward over the front leg. Reach your left hand down and place it on top of the Backbridge. You can keep your head in a neutral position looking at the floor or straight ahead, or begin to move the gaze up to your right hand. Stay here and breathe for 30 seconds and then release the twist on an inhalation to bring your torso back upright. Repeat on the other side.

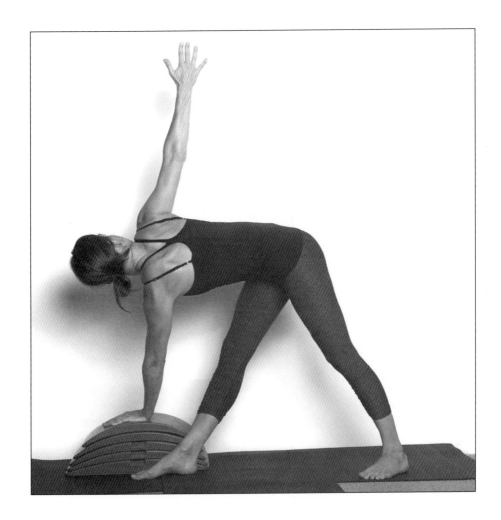

Prasarita Padottanasana (Wide-Legged Forward Bend)

Place the Backbridge in front of you on the ground, with the long edge facing you. Widen your stance approximately 3 feet, with the inner edges of your feet parallel to each other. Place your hands on your hips and inhale while you lift your chest and lengthen your spine. As you exhale, keep a flat back and begin to bend forward at the hips. When your torso is parallel to the floor, place your palms on the Backbridge, fingertips pointing forward. Bend your elbows directly back, bringing your forehead to rest on top of the Backbridge, level 5. For more flexible practitioners, use a lower level. Remain active in your legs and draw your shoulders away from your ears. Stay in the pose for 30 seconds. Slowly rise up until your torso is parallel to the ground and your arms are extended straight under your shoulders. Place your hands back on your hips and slowly rise on an inhale to return to standing.

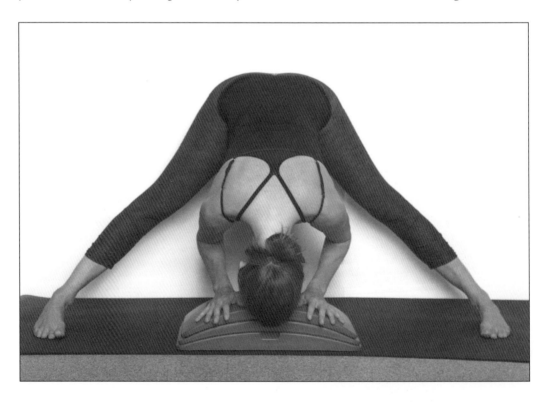

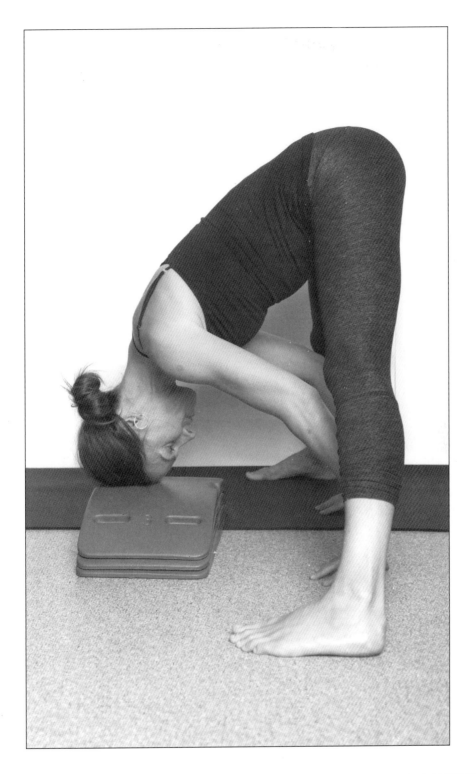

Utthan Pristhasana (Lizard Pose)

Place the Backbridge at the front of your mat with the long edge facing you. Start in downward facing dog. Step your left foot between your hands to a lunge position then move that foot out to the left of the Backbridge. Lower your forearms to the Backbridge inside the left foot. The lower the level of the Backbridge you use, the more intense this hip opener will feel. For advanced practitioners, keep the inner right thigh lifting up and as straight as possible. Novice practitioners can lower the right knee to the mat. As your right heel reaches back, your heart opens forward to create length in your upper back. Breathe in the pose for 30 seconds and then step back to down dog and switch sides. You can also use the Backbridge as padding under your back knee.

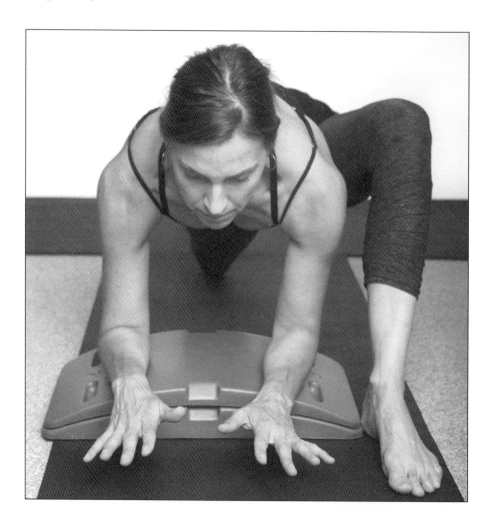

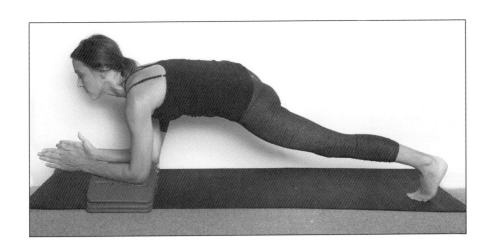

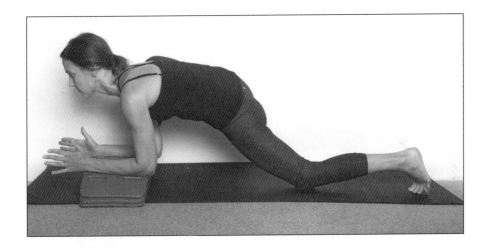

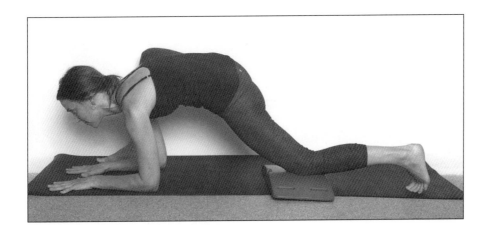

Malasana (Squat)

Place the Backbridge on the mat with the long side facing you. Stand in front of the Backbridge with your feet as wide as your mat. Squat down and sit on the center of the Backbridge, keeping your heels on the mat. More advanced practitioners can use lower levels of the Backbridge while beginners or yogis with tighter hips can use level 4 or 5. Press your elbows against the inside of your knees and press your palms together in front of your chest with your thumbs touching your sternum (chest). Press your elbows back against your knees and raise your chest to lengthen your front body. Stay here and breathe for 30 seconds.

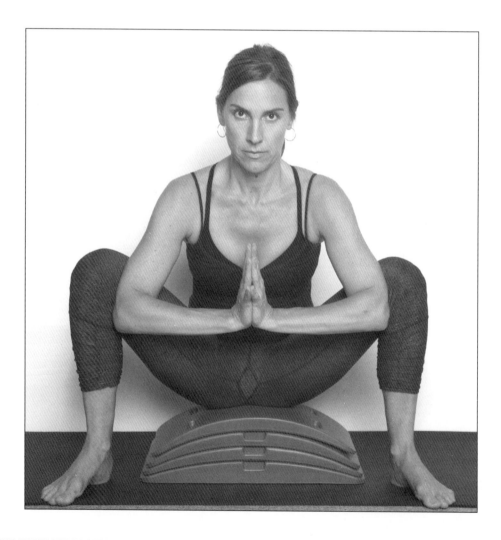

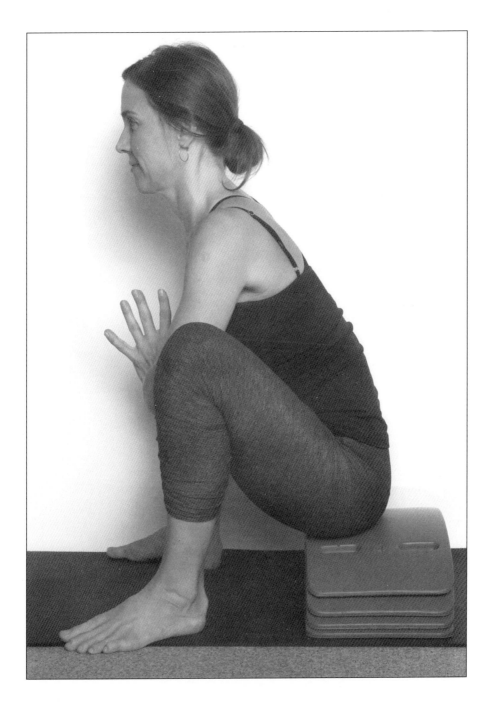

Baddha Konasana (Bound Angle Or Butterfly Pose)

Sit on the Backbridge and bring your feet in as close as possible. Place the soles of the feet together, letting the knees slowly drop open towards the mat. You can gently push down on your thighs with your elbows or on your lower legs with your forearms to increase the stretch. From here, hinge forward at the hips and grasp your feet, maintaining length in the spine.

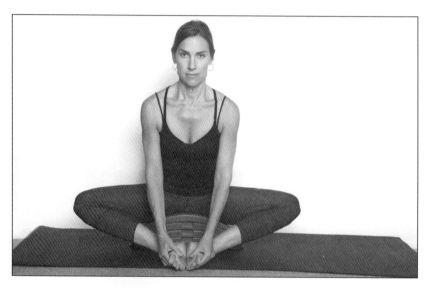

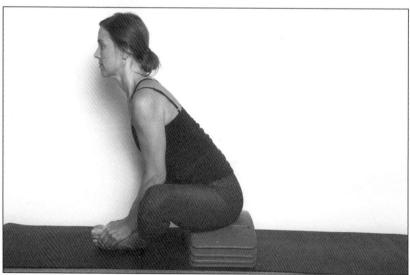

Continue to fold forward over your thighs as far as you can, eventually bringing your fore-head to the ground in front of your feet. Hold for 15-30 seconds.

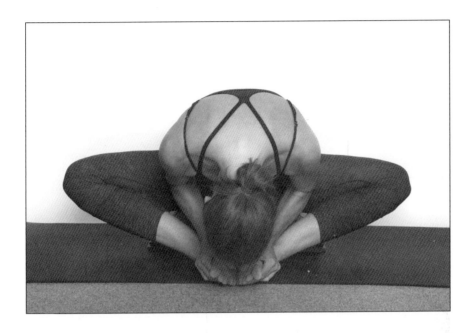

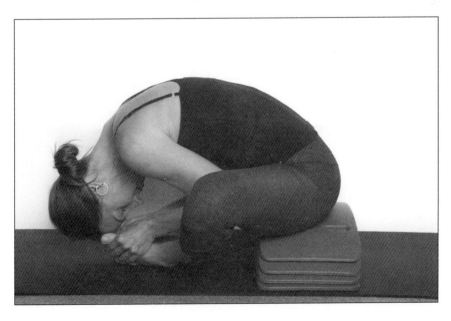

Eka Pada Rajakapotasana
(Pigeon Pose) Sleeping Variation

Come back into pigeon pose. Inhale and lengthen and then exhale and fold forward, lowering your torso on your right thigh for a few breaths. Stretch your arms forward, into sleeping pigeon.

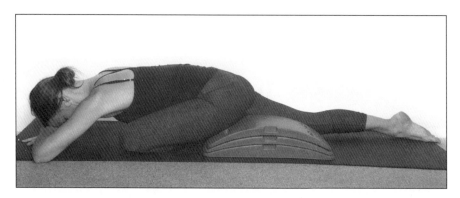

You can also try a twist in this sleeping pigeon pose by twisting your torso and bringing the back of your right shoulder to the mat underneath you. Place your left arm on top of your extended right arm and put your right cheek on the mat. Breathe here for 15-30 seconds. Slowly return to tabletop and repeat pigeon on the other side. The Backbridge allows the hips to stay neutral and grounded in the pose, keeping the integrity of your alignment and allowing those with tight hips to better feel the stretch.

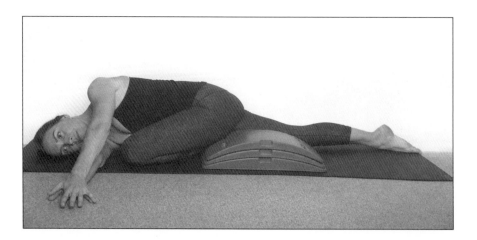

Dandasana (Staff Pose)

Sit on the Backbridge levels 1, 2 or 3 and stretch both legs out in front of you, making sure you sit up straight with a long spine. You can place your fingertips on the floor on either side of you. This pose lengthens the spine and is important to do before forward bends or between poses (especially twists), as it helps return the spine to neutral. The Backbridge changes the angle of the hips in this pose, enabling yogis with tight hips to more easily sit up straight.

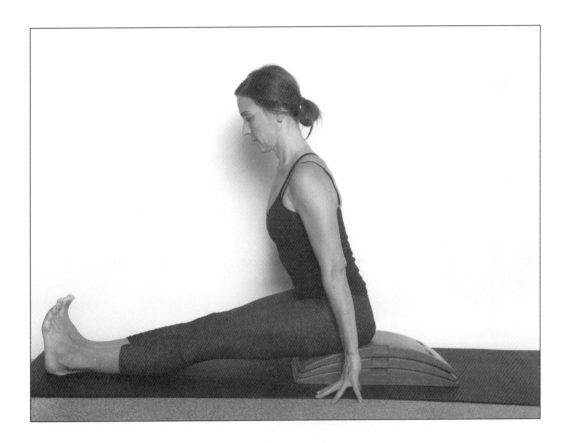

Paschimottanasana (Seated Forward Bend)

From Dadasana, lean forward, maintaining a flat back, and bend at the hips, reaching your hands to grab your shins, ankles or toes. The stretch strap can help you if you are not able to reach.

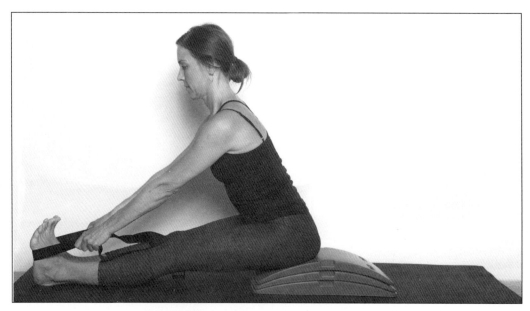

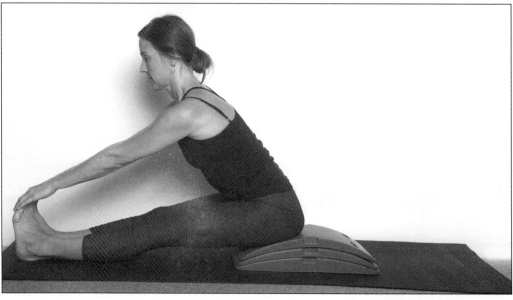

For those practitioners who wish to go further, continue to fold forward until your torso rests on your thighs and your forehead rests on your knees or shins.

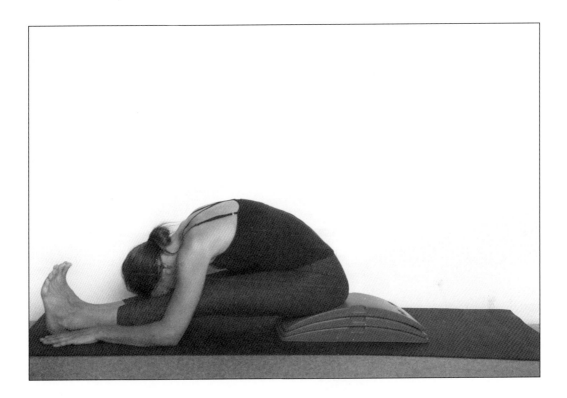

Janu Sirsasana (Head-To-Knee Forward Bend)

Sit perpendicular on levels 1, 2 or 3 of the Backbridge and place one leg out straight in front of you. Bend your other knee and bring the sole of your foot to the inner thigh of your outstretched leg. Bend at the hips and lean forward with a straight back, reaching for the ankle of your outstretched leg. You may also use a strap. Hold the pose for several breaths and repeat on the other side.

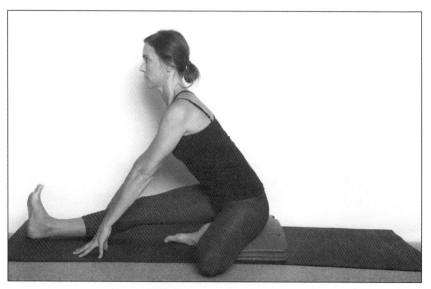

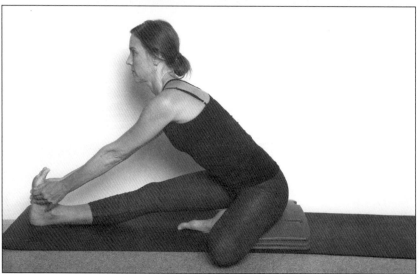

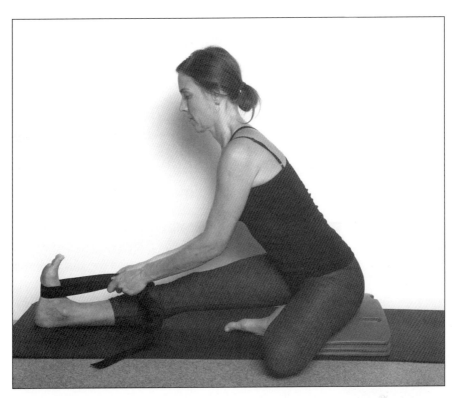

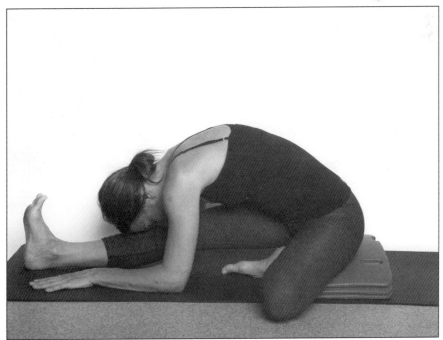

Marichyasana III (Marichi's Pose) and Marichyasana I (Pose Dedicated to the Sage Marichi, I)

Sit in Dandasana and bend your right knee, placing your foot on the floor so that your heel is as close to your right sitting bone as possible. Keep your left leg active, pressing into the floor with the foot flexed. With a straight arm, place your right hand on the mat behind the Backbridge. Bending your left arm, twist your torso to the right and place the outside of your left elbow on the outside of your right knee. Inhale and lengthen your torso. Exhale and twist more to the right. Repeat for several breaths and then return to center.

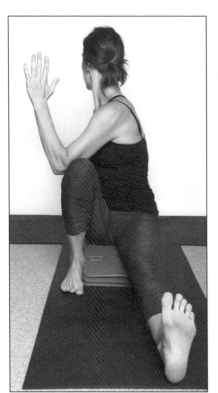
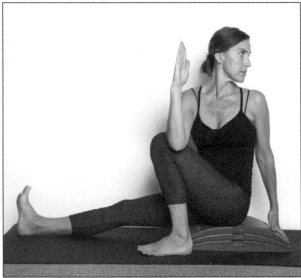

Now, reach your arms forward and grab the toes of your outstretched leg. If you can't reach, using the stretch strap can help you still get a deep stretch.

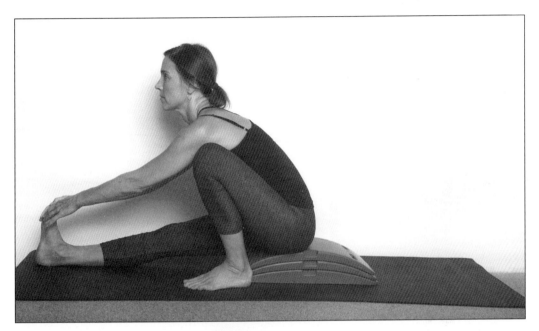

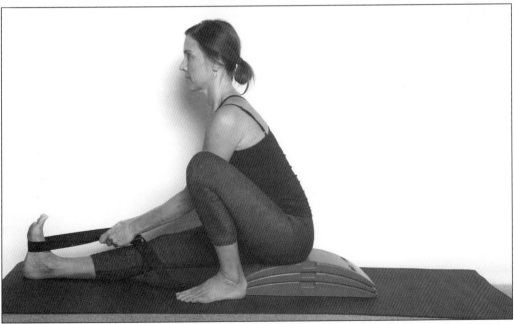

Rotate your arm so your right thumb points to the floor and the palm faces out to the right. As you reach your arm forward, lengthen your torso forward as well. From here, bring the right arm back around the knee, reaching the right hand to the outside of the right thigh or buttock. Sweep your left arm behind your low back and grab your right wrist in your left hand. If you cannot reach, use a strap. Once you have the bind, inhale to lengthen your spine and draw the shoulders away from your ears. Exhale to gently lower your torso as close as possible to the top of your left leg. Hold here for several breaths and then release the bind and return to sitting. Repeat with opposite leg.

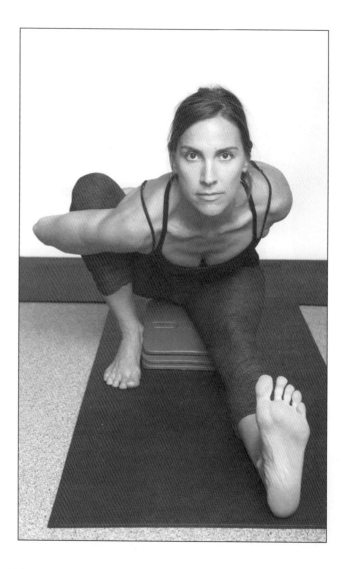

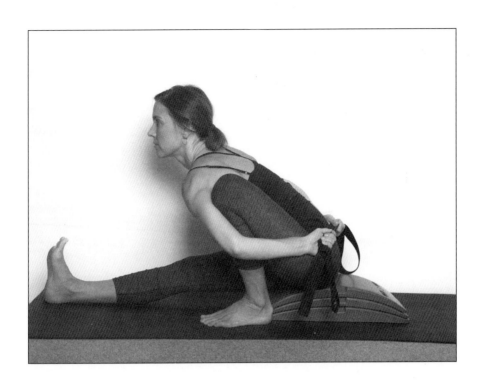

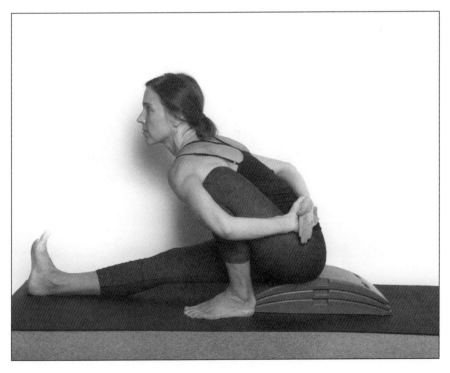

Ardha Virasana (Half Hero)

Sit on the Backbridge levels 2 or 3 and place one leg out straight. Take your other leg and bend it, bringing your shin in underneath your thigh with the top of the foot on the mat. The Backbridge will allow you to comfortably sit and stretch in this position without hurting your bent knee. With a straight back, bend at the hip and lean forward, reaching for the ankle of your outstretched leg. If you have tight hamstrings, this can also be done with the stretch strap. Repeat on the other side.

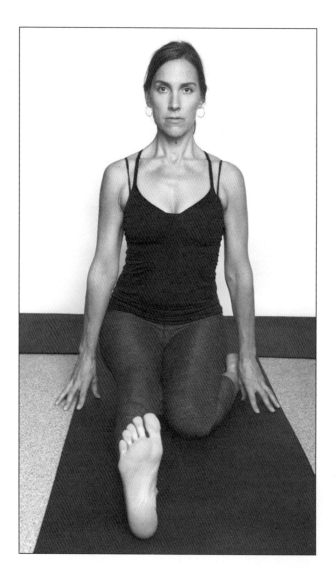

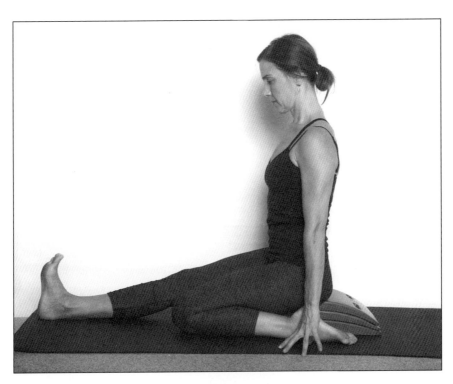

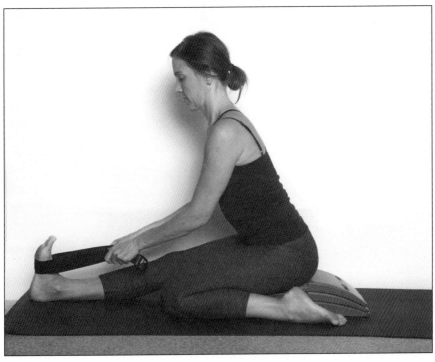

Hanumanasana (Monkey Pose Or Split)

Kneel on the floor with the Backbridge parallel to and just in front of your knees. Step your right foot forward in front of the Backbridge and rotate your right thigh out, peeling the sole of your right foot off the floor. With your fingertips on the floor on either side of the Backbridge, lean slightly forward while you slowly slide your left knee back, straightening the leg and lowering your right buttock towards the top of the Backbridge. From here you can extend the right heel away from your torso, gradually turning your leg as it straightens to bring your right kneecap to point up toward the ceiling. As your front leg straightens, continue extending your left knee back with the left kneecap pointing toward the floor, carefully lowering the top of the left thigh and the back of the right leg and buttocks to the Backbridge. Beginning practitioners can use a higher level of the Backbridge for support in this pose. Breathe here for 15-30 seconds. To come out of the pose, press your hands into the floor and turn your right leg out slightly as you slowly return your right heel and your left knee to their starting positions. Reverse the legs and repeat.

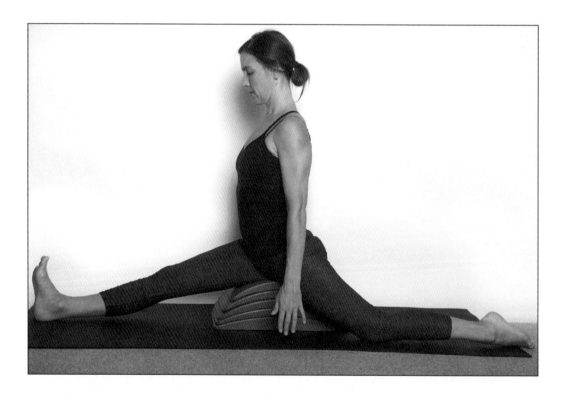

Supta Virasana (Reclining Hero Pose)

From Hero pose (p. 194), move the Backbridge behind you so that you are sitting just in front of the short edge. Begin to lower your back toward the Backbridge by leaning onto your hands, then your forearms and elbows. Novice practitioners may remain here or continue reclining onto the Backbridge. The higher levels of the Backbridge will generate a more intense back bend, but will create less pressure in the knees. You can rest your hands on the backs of your heels or angle them out on the sides of your torso, palms up. Stay in this pose for up to 2 minutes.

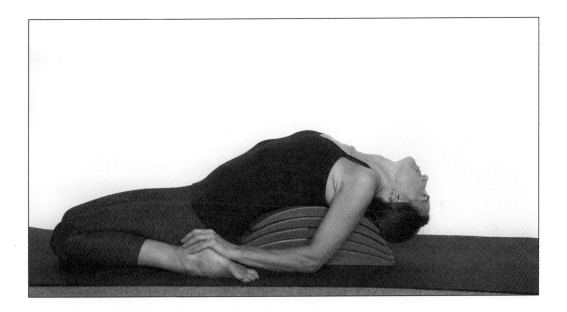

Setu Bandha Sarvangasana (Bridge Pose)

Lie on your back with your buttocks resting just below the highest point of the Backbridge. Bend your knees and put your feet on the floor with your heels close to the end of the Backbridge. Your arms should lay flat on either side of you. Level 5 provides the most support for beginners. You can rest here without lifts for a supported, restorative version of bridge pose. As you progress, lower the level of your Backbridge. Keeping your thighs and inner feet parallel, press your feet and arms into the floor as you lift your buttocks off the Backbridge until your thighs are nearly parallel to the floor. Stay here for 15-30 seconds and gently release by rolling the spine slowly down onto the Backbridge. Repeat 2-3 times.

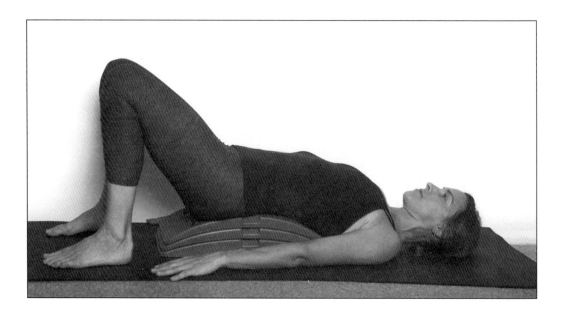

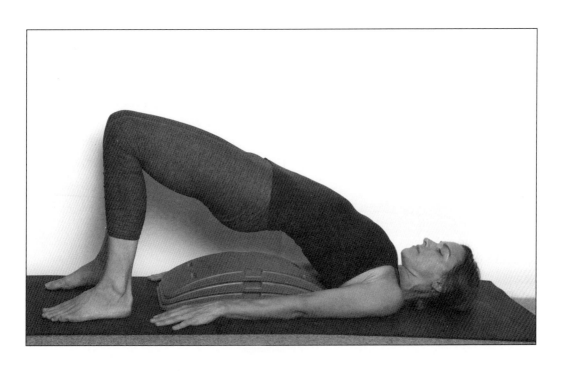

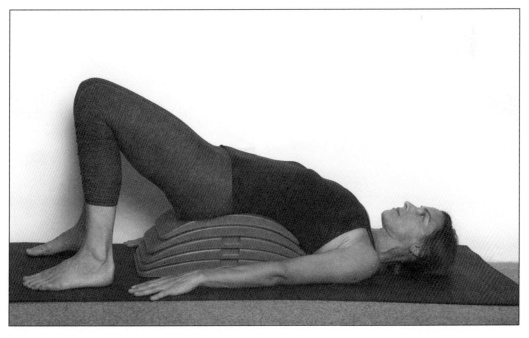

Reclining Twist

Lie flat on your back and place the Backbridge about 12 inches to the side of your hips. Keep your shoulders flat on the mat and bring one knee towards your chest. With the other leg flat on the mat, pull your bent leg across your torso, placing it on the Backbridge. You may place your opposite hand on top of the bent knee, applying gentle downward pressure to increase the stretch. Hold for 15-30 seconds and repeat on the opposite side. Try different levels of the Backbridge to find which is most comfortable for you (level 1 will give the biggest stretch.)

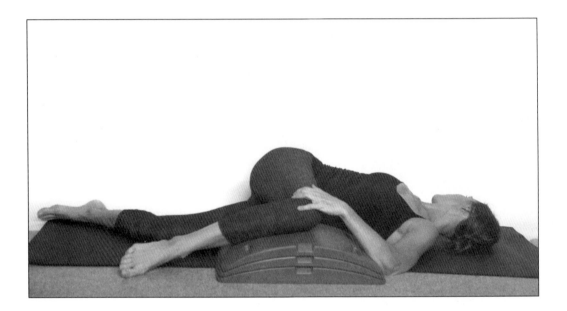

Supta Baddha Konasana (Reclining Bound Angle Pose)

Sit in front of the Backbridge with your buttocks just touching the short end. Take Baddha Konasana pose by pulling your feet in as close as possible. Place the soles of the feet together, letting the knees gently drop open towards the mat. Slowly recline back over the Backbridge, letting your arms drape to the sides, palms up or down, and with your head resting on the mat. Hold for 30 seconds to 1 minute. The higher levels of the Backbridge will give a deeper backbend for more advanced practitioners.

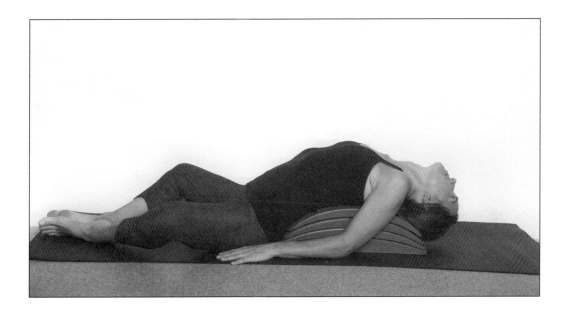

CONCLUSION

A Stretch a Day for a Balanced Body

After seeing countless patients suffering from back pain caused by too much forward flexion, I designed the Backbridge as a simple way to stretch the back by putting extension into one's spine. The Backbridge extension stretch can both cure and stave off future back pain associated by many structural causes if done daily and is truly revolutionary despite its simplicity. As I experimented further with the Backbridge, I was thrilled to find that it offers so many more applications and benefits to the entire body. I consider *The Ultimate Backbridge Stretch Book* to be the best medication and prevention for countless injuries and physical complaints, including tightness, muscle pain, and even sprains and strains. It has been deliberately designed for people of all levels to use and tailor to their individual needs. Sampling the different stretches and routines will help you identify which areas of your body need the most attention. Remember, all of us should be doing some stretching regularly to keep us not only loose and limber, but also free of core imbalance. I urge you to get creative, using the Backbridge as a tool to assist in stretching your entire body. Show it to your yoga teacher and bring it along to the gym to help spread the word about this helpful stretching tool, and I bet you'll have others thanking you!

As you are stretching using your Backbridge and this book, remember this: The Backbridge can be extremely therapeutic as well as diagnostic. Listen to your body and observe where you are feeling tight or stiff in a particular stretch. Back pain may actually be coming from tight hips or hamstrings. Spend extra time gently working those areas using the stretches I designated for those body parts and see if you notice a change, both in that particular local area and in your back!

Don't let the Backbridge's simple looking design fool you. Some exercises or poses in the book can be quite intense, so please do not over stretch and always use a level of the Backbridge that best suits your body. Over time, you will notice that your flexibility will dramatically improve and the Backbridge can safely guide you through the advanced stretches in this book.

Realigning your spine and improving your posture and flexibility are some of the most important things that you can do for your health. Backbridge stretching should become part of your daily routine because it can really have a lasting impact on the quality of your life. If you don't have the time for a longer routine, just make sure that you are at least doing the Backbridge spinal extension stretch for approximately two minutes in the morning and two minutes in the evening. I'm not sure if the phrase "An apple a day keeps the doctor away" is true, but in this case, one stretch a day most certainly can help keep your entire body aligned and balanced and help you avoid many more invasive treatments—even surgery!

If you are interested in more information about the Backbridge, I have created several other resources with additional research on this important product. Please refer to my book *Three Weeks to A Better Back*, which explores the many structural, nutritional and emotional issues that can contribute to back pain and offers a multitude of solutions based on your individual diagnosis. You can also visit backbridge.com for tool-specific information or go to my website, DrSinett.com, for article-based research.

Wishing you the best of health, and happy stretching!

Dr. Todd Sinett

ACKNOWLEDGMENTS

Firstly, I'd like to thank my patients, who have unwittingly served as my test cases and allowed me to grow both personally and professionally. I want to thank the engineering marvels at FactorsNY who gave someone, who had never created anything in his life before, the opportunity to create an amazingly simple yet tremendously helpful product. To my beautiful wife and my children: thank you for your continued support as I continue to take time to explore medicine and improve my practice. May you all stay flexible in the rigors of life. I want to thank my publisher Pauline at East End Press for believing in what I have to say, and my amazing editor Jayne Pillemer who takes every decent idea I have and makes it intelligent. Thank you to Tasman Rubel, who not only manages my Manhattan wellness center but also all of my work endeavors with pure genius. I want to thank my fitness models, Alexandra Torres and Stephanie Culen, for their insight and flexibility. I would like to especially honor the memory of David Zanes and express my gratitude for the beautiful photographs he took for this book. Thank you to my late father, Sheldon Sinett DC, who taught me to never just accept a patient's pain and to really look for unique solutions in an effort to continually better our healthcare. I want to thank my mother for her never-ending encouragement. Lastly, thank you to the readers of this book. I really hope the information in it helps you achieve greater flexibility, balance and overall improved function in your life.

INDEX OF STRETCHES, BALANCES AND POSES